Caregiving

The Spiritual Journey
of Love, Loss, and Renewal

Beth Witrogen McLeod

John Wiley & Sons, Inc.

New York • Chichester • Weinheim • Brisbane • Singapore • Toronto

This book is printed on acid-free paper. ♾

Copyright © 1999 by Beth Witrogen McLeod. All rights reserved
Published by John Wiley & Sons, Inc.
Published simultaneously in Canada

The author gratefully acknowedges permission to use the following:
"I saw grief," from *Birdsong: 53 Short Poems*, by Rumi, translated by Coleman Barks.
© 1993, Coleman Barks, Maypop. Excerpt from "The Caregivers," by Beth Witrogen
McLeod. © 1995, *The San Francisco Examiner*. Excerpts from *Complaints of a Dutiful
Daughter*. © 1994, Deborah Hoffmann.

This publication is designed to provide accurate and authoritative information in regard to
the subject matter covered. It is sold with the understanding that the publisher is not
engaged in rendering professional services. If professional advice
or other expert assistance is required, the services of a competent professional
person should be sought.

Library of Congress Cataloging-in-Publication Data:

McLeod, Beth Witrogen
    Caregiving : the spiritual journey of love, loss, and renewal / Beth Witrogen McLeod.
    p.   cm.
    Includes bibliographical references and index.
    ISBN 0-471-25408-8 (hardcover : alk. paper)
    1. Terminal care. 2. Caregivers. 3. Bereavement—Psychological aspects. I. Title.
R726.8.M39 1994
362.1'75—dc21   98-41472
                                         CIP

Printed in the United States of America

10 9 8 7 6 5 4 3 2 1

For my parents,
Mel and Elaine Witrogen,
and for my husband, Bob McLeod,
the three who gave me life

Contents

Acknowledgments

Like caregiving, writing a book feels solitary, but no one truly accomplishes it alone. Every person who has shared a painful or happy story, everyone who encouraged me both during my parents' illnesses and my long journey back, helped create this book.

But some people must be recognized by name: foremost is my husband, Bob, without whose lovingkindness, wisdom, humor, patience, and generosity of spirit I would have stayed forever submerged; the indomitable Samantha Ko; my agents, Laurie Fox and Linda Chester, whose faith and support honor the soul in us all; my editor at John Wiley & Sons, Thomas Miller, whose insightful and caring work greatly enhanced the evolution and substance of this work; my sister, Marcia, for her willingness; Anne Bashkiroff, Claudine Michael, Tom Scott, Bob Knight, Ray Denton, Hospice Inc., Tammy and Ken Breeden, Faye Johnson, Cleo Houston, Erma Garnes, Marcia and Buzz Solomon, Beverly Jacobson, Leslie Innes, P. S. Thorne; the *Wichita Eagle*; and Steve Cook and other friends at the *San Francisco Examiner* who supported my series, "The Caregivers," and understood the need to follow my heart.

Especially I extend humble, deep appreciation to the hundred-plus caregivers who so openly shared such intimate pain; and to the approximately one hundred professionals who graciously lent expertise. I am indebted to the hundreds of other caregivers who have participated in my weekly AOL caregiver support chat; their stories form the heart of *Caregiving*. I am also indebted to the Alzheimer's e-mail group for their trust and inspiration.

To respect the wishes of caregivers who requested anonymity, their names have been changed—but not their tales, all of which validate this life passage as a spiritual journey. I regret the inability to print everyone's story, because each is valuable. No comment, no outpouring, no experience has been without meaning: all bear witness to family caregivers everywhere, and to the heroic nature of caring itself.

Note from the author

If you have a caregiving story to share, or comments about *Caregiving,* write Beth Witrogen McLeod, c/o John Wiley & Sons, Inc., 605 Third Avenue, New York, NY 10158, or witrogen@ccnet.com for email correspondence.

Introduction

The other night I had this dream:

> *I am rushing to catch a train but have forgotten some valuables at the hotel. When I return, I find the room unlocked and all my belongings stolen. Weeping uncontrollably, I run to rescue the one prize I had carefully hidden: my late parents' jewelry box, filled with the exquisite pieces that are my sole inheritance. But it is not there.*
>
> *As others try to comfort me, I tell them that everything of importance is gone. No one understands the depth of my loss; there can be no consolation. Yet as I wander weakly around the room, I discover that the thieves dropped the container, now empty. On impulse I turn it upside down and notice a secret compartment I never knew existed. Inside are boxes my father has carefully wrapped, like tiny presents, each containing large uncut stones of impossible value.*
>
> *My parents have provided for me in my moment of deepest anguish: knowledge that we all contain the potential to shine richly and to reflect outwardly the spirit that yearns within. It is up to each of us to take that journey to wholeness—then manifest it in service to others.*

I never saw it coming. I was drifting blithely along in my tidy little life, as naive and immortal as the next fortysomething. Suddenly both my parents were catastrophically ill, and my life was abruptly derailed. Everything that had been familiar vanished; what might come was terrifyingly uncertain.

The initial severing came the instant my father informed me, over aching distance at the end of my work day at the *San Francisco Examiner*, that my mother had amyotrophic lateral sclerosis, not arthritis. He could not speak the "D" word; he didn't have to. His own life was already on the line after a fifth and final surgery to remove another grapefruit-sized tumor from the hollow that had once housed his tailbone.

My father's words, delivered lightly in his desire to protect me, shattered my childhood, stole my future, and undermined the security that had cloistered me until that moment: my identity as a daughter, my parents' little girl, someone who would be shielded from life's vicissitudes by the two people who would always care. In their illnesses they suffered greatly, a relentless ricocheting from crisis to crisis in pain and misfortune. And when they were long past all possibility of remaining in their home, my parents were packed up and shuttled to a convalescent facility where they later died, five weeks apart, nearly bankrupt from medical bills and invisible after decades of public service.

In some ways they never knew what hit them; in some ways neither did I, not until long after they passed and I had time, and energy, to reflect on all that had transpired. Despite the best of intentions and arguments to the contrary, I never felt I did enough for them.

Their fate changed my life forever. Grief is still my adviser; sometimes it is a friend and reminds me of my humble place in the universe, opening life to the mysterious gifts of awe and gratitude. At other times it casts me down and turns my heart to stone. In the best of times I know loss to be merely a matter of perspective; in the worst I lose my soul to anger at life's brief luminescence.

Who Are the Caregivers?

My parents left a double-edged legacy: awareness of both the sorrow and the generosity of the human heart. Nowhere perhaps is this paradox more widely played out than on the daily stage of family caregiving, where the unsuspecting can find themselves on a chaotic journey in which the only certainty is the demise of their loved one. These caregivers are on a path seemingly without end, subjected to the stresses and the guilts of watching another's pain without being able to erase it, of witnessing a loved one's dying without being able to prevent it. They quietly sacrifice personal agendas to look after those in need, often sandwiched between child care and jobs and usually without advance planning. They live a world apart from everyday reality and wonder if they will ever be normal again. They have one goal: to maintain the dignity and the well-being of their loved one until the end. The burden is great, the information insufficient, the doubt overpowering. Yet these loyal souls—many of whom do not recognize themselves as caregivers—work largely without professional help, feeling they can and must do everything alone. There is no question about taking on this role: they do so compelled not only by the dictates of society, but also by the mandates of the heart.

They bathe, feed, dress, shop for, listen to, and transport frail parents, spouses, children, friends, relatives, neighbors, and even strangers. Night and day they torment over how to keep loved ones out of nursing homes, how to give adequate medical attention and make life-and-death decisions when they have not been trained to do so. Often in poor health or over age sixty-five themselves, they worry about safeguarding an obstinate relative's finances or moving him or her to a more secure home.

They are the parents who lovingly tend to disabled children. They are the grandparents raising grandkids because their own children are incarcerated, divorced, or on drugs. They are the well spouses who grieve while their mates still live but have forgotten all the love that ever passed between them. They are the adult children who have discovered an entirely new and unanticipated midlife crisis: caring for an aging parent. They are mostly women.

In individual ways they blaze their own trails and build support networks. Each caregiver must deal with challenges like handling complex medical and legal documents, finding appropriate housing or care facilities, modifying a home for safety, moving a loved one cross-country, massaging a child forever confined to bed, or changing the diaper on a modest and humiliated parent. Loved ones who have been independent now fear becoming burdensome; family patterns are turned upside down and futures forever altered. Usually these tasks are carried out with courage and persistence against frustrating odds. Shorn of energy but loyal and loving to the end, family caregivers more than measure up to the demands: they are stalwarts who persevere against great obstacles.

Caregiving is as much, if not more, about the emotional impact as it is the physical. Long after proper housing or medical care has been arranged, greater personal issues remain: How do we keep·our hearts open in hell? And why should we try? This is the inner journey of caregiving; this is the promise of renewal.

"Caregivers are ordinary people caught up in extraordinary events," says Daniel Paris, a geriatric social worker at Massachusetts General Hospital in Boston. Although family caregiving has always existed across all cultural and economic settings, some elements are unique to this era: an increasingly aged and disabled population that will be fueled by the massive baby boom generation now entering midlife, the lack of adequate and coordinated systems to finance and support long-term care of the chronically ill and disabled, and a renaissance in spiritual seeking and exploration of end-of-life issues.

Along with global graying, we have entered what geriatric experts call the "third age," the extension of healthy middle age well into what used to be known as the sunset years. Until the Industrial Revolution, only one in ten people could expect to live to sixty-five. Today most will reach that age—and well beyond. Though most elderly are healthier than ever, it is a time when the ravages of oldest age require the most support services. In North America, the number of family caregivers has exploded by 300 percent in only nine years, reaching into a quarter of all households: the most pressing long-term need of the chronically ill is not skilled nursing but help with daily activities such as grooming or getting out of bed.

The personal stories in *Caregiving* profile those who care for our aging, ill, and disabled and the lengths they travel in health care systems trying to control long-term-care costs while living in a society that idolizes youth and independence rather than wisdom and community.

The Spirit of Caregiving

Caregiving reveals how assuming the care of a dependent loved one has the potential to alter us at the core of our being, opening our heart's capacity to live fully even in the midst of loss. Because our death-denying society has few safety nets for coping with suffering, caregiving often hits people unprepared to negotiate the raw emotions that underlie our identities, our relationships, and our spiritual beliefs. When those unfamiliar feelings surface, we are unprotected by what we have been conditioned to expect, unaware of the anchor that lies within. When illness, death, and loss find us, we discover some shocking truths: we have not made authentic connections with others, including family, we don't know ourselves well; and we do not feel empowered by the institutions in which we have put our trust.

While I was caring for my parents, I fought to find meaning in suffering. After my caregiving days were over and colleagues began to experience the throes of parent care, they asked me how I survived. The answer, I found, was in looking at caregiving as a spiritual practice. I discovered countless clues in the journeys described by mystics and shamans as well as in classic mythological and wisdom traditions that reveal suffering as a path to liberation if viewed as a spiritual discipline. These teachings frame *Caregiving* to provide an accessible, workable guide through this dreaded labyrinth.

Although the subjects of illness and death may be uncomfortable, the tales herein provide support and comfort: knowledge that we are not alone, that we have choice and permission, and that there is a way out of confusion. Caregiver stories, interviews with professionals and spiritual leaders, and literary references give strategies for addressing the two most difficult emotional issues: coping with the stresses of caring for a loved one and moving forward with so much loss.

Exploring the spiritual dimension of end-of-life issues, this book charts family caregiving as a rite of passage. Taken as a soul's journey, it is an everyday path with heart, a way to attend to the practical details while also fulfilling our essential nature. When grief strips us of superficial relationships and dreams, what we have left is true connectedness as witnessed through the ages. In Christianity's crucifixion and resurrection, in shamanic tales of initiation, in Buddhist doctrines of compassion, the message has always been that who we are *not* changes; who we truly *are* is eternal and compelled to help relieve suffering.

This path mirrors the archetypal mythical adventure in which the seeker is called to action and descends to a mysterious inner world where latent strengths come forth to guide him home again, wiser and more mature. This unwelcome territory is described in classic theological mysticism as the dark night of the soul, a calling to change predictable behaviors in order to fulfill a higher purpose. Transformation happens at the bottommost point of despair, an initiation into larger life aided by others who have learned the way out and appear when help is most needed.

Incorporating these lessons leads to a richer appreciation of life and is one of the promises of mindful caregiving. To help realize that potential, *Caregiving* is structured to offer companionship on whatever level the reader needs, from practical to spiritual. Although fullest benefit will be derived by reading the book from beginning to end, each chapter is constructed to be self-containing.

Navigating the inner journey from personal crisis to the awakened heart of compassion, *Caregiving* is interwoven by my personal story. Part I, Setting Out on the Path of Caregiving, explores family and communication dynamics, when to become involved, women's issues, the medical and financial maze, and parent and spousal care. Part II, Emotional Wilderness, examines the nature of loss, stress and anxiety, depression, and hitting bottom. Part III, Bridges to the Future, lays out the strategies and everyday miracles that span the old life and the new, such as support groups, professional help, alternative medicine, and religious traditions. End-of-life issues are also presented in this rite of passage. Part IV, Reclaiming Life, proposes a new vision of relationship, aging, and community. Where appropriate, action steps are suggested to help chart the way.

Doomsayers would preach that the world has been overtaken by rage, greed, and resignation. I believe that if you look into the private rooms of caregiving families, you will find the true nature of things as they are, beneath the veneer of social conditioning and confusion, stereotype and illusion. There you will find great kindness and devotion, a trust of life that surpasses doubt or pain. There you will find the highest expression of who we are.

If we close our hearts to suffering, we cannot open them to love. Every benevolent act counts. By surviving difficulties and holding on to goodness, caregivers inspire others to summon the power of the spirit. Humanity *can* evolve from its violence and recklessness into an enlightened age of caring when the lessons of loss are honored, exemplified by modern-day heroes who fulfill the age-old mandate: to give.

My Parents Are Dying

When the phone call came that September evening, the news broadsided me so completely I have never returned to the person I was. That life was destroyed the moment I had to face the mortality of a parent.

"Doll," my dad said with so much sweetness, "Mommy doesn't have arthritis. She has Lou Gehrig's disease." Time stood still. Nothing that had been real was true any longer; nothing I had counted on could ever be certain again. A major life change had just been announced: terminal illness not of just one parent but now of two, twelve hundred miles away. For thirty years Father had triumphed over a rare, recurrent cancer, losing some functions but never his spirit. Over those years it was my resilient mother who breezed through every emergency, who continually said, "I'm not worried"—the one who was always there, the one who would always be there.

My father, Mel, had always insisted he was more than the sum of his illnesses. He lived as if he were immortal—so naturally we who loved him assumed he was. For decades he and my mother, Elaine, had been pillars of their Kansas city, instrumental in helping build Wichita's civic, artistic, educational, medical, and religious institutions while mediating in community relations. My mother was known both for her kindness and for her love of the arts: a music prodigy, she received a Steinway baby grand at the age of ten when her parents had it trucked from New York to Oklahoma.

Against this backdrop it was inconceivable that my parents could die, certainly not like this. My innocent belief—that doing all the right things guaranteed immortality—was most decimated by the unwelcome truth that the woman who had given me birth was dying. I immediately lost all bearing—my faith, anchor, and direction—before death's reality.

Mother had been showing symptoms of the disease for months—possibly years—but we had failed to notice much beyond a slight loss of energy and memory. It seems we had a habit of not noticing my mother, who was becoming more persistent in her need for attention. We decided to get a second opinion from a recommended neurologist at the University of California Medical Center in San Francisco.

Dad thought I should be with my reluctant mother in the examining rooms. First came the shock of seeing her once-rounded body already atrophied. There she was, crying out in pain from tests for muscle strength in one room, covering up for memory loss in a second, and in yet another, darkened room, mournfully looking up at me from the table as they pricked her with needles, trying to be good to her, analyzing the telltale wave on the monitor. She kept telling the technician she'd always been a piano teacher, as if he cared; but she still cared as she clung desperately to her past, to her proud identity disappearing now with every snap of a neuron coming to its end.

She was overwhelmed, she was frightened, and we didn't speak of it. We didn't want her to suffer with the knowledge of her death, and so she suffered alone.

PART I

Setting Out on the Path of Caregiving

CHAPTER I

What Family Caregiving Is

I saw grief drinking a cup of sorrow
and called out,
          "It tastes sweet,
does it not?"
          "You've caught me,"
grief answered,
          "and you've ruined my business.
How can I sell sorrow,
          when you know it's a blessing?"— Rumi

For some it comes like a bump in the night; for others, it is a realization of having already been swept away. We become caregivers by choice, by default, and by obligation; we assume the role because the alternatives are unacceptable. In a culture defined by short attention spans and sound bites, family caregiving demands investment for the long term, often an abrogation of dreams and a wholesale reconstruction of the future, one slow brick at a time.

Caregiving—the act of providing assistance to someone ill or frail— is emerging from the modest recesses of everyday life into one of the most catalytic challenges any of us will face. Even when families have made preparations for possible disability, it is the unanticipated events—a fall, a stroke, a creeping inability to maintain a checkbook—that define the turning point from a life so familiar to one filled with incalculable unknowns.

The typical informal caregiver is an employed forty-six-year-old woman who works another eighteen hours a week caring for her mother. The typical recipient is a seventy-seven-year-old woman who lives nearby but alone and has at least one chronic condition, such as heart disease or osteoporosis. Despite myths to the contrary, families do not abandon their loved ones to institutions when they become chronically or terminally ill. Most are cared for at home, in their communities, at all costs.

Family caregiving is an emotional roller coaster that can leave a person exhausted, bewildered, and dislodged, wondering how she or he can feel so helpless in a period so supposedly grown-up. Each stage of an illness presents a succession of hurdles, stretching hearts more than it seems possible to bear. At times it would be enough just to hear, "You're doing a good job," but even that reinforcement can be elusive.

Because most people are reluctant to ask for help or to admit they may be in trouble, caregivers can face obstacles merely in sorting out what the problems are. Often there is only a sense of something amiss: a hesitant phrase, increased isolation. Adult children suddenly must pry out of secretive or distrustful parents the most private of details about estate matters; spouses who have never made decisions now must make all of them. Parents may have divorced or been unloving; siblings or relatives may have vanished at the first spot of trouble. For young adults who couldn't wait to leave the parental yoke, time and distance now complicate the best intentions and hide the worst scenarios. Few people want to think about death, let alone plan for it. The lucky ones discover that their parents or spouses have already seen to legal documents, health insurance, and funeral arrangements. For others, the discovery phase can be a long ride into purgatory.

Dwayne, now fifty-two, had been a high school athlete. He was doted on by his mother, Marthe, who labored thirty-one hours to birth him and who later sacrificed so that he could have the education, even the foods, he wanted. When he asked to attend his dream high school, she got a clerk's job to make it happen. When he wanted to take on a paper route, she encouraged him to be a kid as long as possible. During his trips home from college, Marthe would stay up late into the night, soaking up every story, supporting her son's decision to go into the Peace Corps after graduation, reveling in his independence.

"Everything I am proud of having done or stood for I owe to my mother and father," says Dwayne. So when Marthe suffered a major stroke that left her blind and partially paralyzed, it was only natural that he would bring her cross-country to live with him, alternating care with his sister, Marlene. Marthe felt it wasn't fair, it wasn't right, that her children should have to give up their lives and finances to take care of her. But a nursing home was unthinkable.

"They said I would be a vegetable," Marthe recalled of the hospital diagnosis. But Dwayne tickled her feet, and sure enough a toe moved. That's when they thought Marthe might have a chance to regain her health. In a relentless pursuit of self-education, Dwayne studied physical, mental, and emotional exercises and the foods and alternative therapies, such as acupuncture, that might strengthen and heal her. Although it meant cutting back on his computer career and social life, Dwayne was glad to do it. He led his mother through intense physical therapy, made her take walks and eat health foods even though Marthe insisted she hated all of it. He built a ballet barre in his living room, rounded up makeshift exercise equipment, and worked with her, like a coach one-on-one, encouraging, prodding, reveling in the little progresses that began to add up to better sight and the ability to walk.

"I was raised a jock, so all this was second nature to me. But she's not from that generation—she doesn't even like exercise—so we would argue for hours. She called me an 'exercise Gestapo.'" Still she obeyed, she trusted, and she improved. They joked and teased as they took their walks, and Marthe pushed the grocery cart for even more exercise. They talked about Dwayne's father, who had died five years earlier, and reminisced about the good times growing up in Ohio. Dwayne's world revolved around his parents' goodness and repaying their kindness. It was a huge balancing act, but he would not let up.

"Pushing Ma to exercise, to think positively, to laugh, to fight her crying jags that struck thirty to forty times on some days gave her back some independence," says Dwayne, who devoted almost six years to it before Marthe passed away. His health deteriorated, his emotions were spent, and he felt guilty for not taking her full time.

Marthe may have resisted the role change, but never the love. Dwayne says: "You get more human the older you get. Part of me says I don't want to forget there's something so special when I think of my mom, something almost holy. I don't want to forget even the last moments. I just wish I had more confidence that I did enough."

The Call to Care

To become a caregiver, we must cross a threshold whose other side is unexplored and often threatening. We may be in denial about warning signs—poor grooming or eating habits, forgetfulness—that foreshadow a change in our lifestyle and focus. We may expect one-time answers for an ever-changing landscape, single solutions for progressive conditions. And we are not yet aware that most health care services are not geared to long-term illness but to prevention and cure.

When do we step in? Unless there is a medical emergency, these are gray areas. There are different levels of care, depending on whether the need is acute, as with a broken bone; chronic, as with a long-term disability; or terminal, which can be short- or long-term. The answer also depends on relationships, family history, communication, honesty, perceptions, fears, and expectations. Conversation may not enhance communication, so it is important to clarify these issues:

~ Am I listening to what the care receiver is expressing through words or body language?
~ Will I appear greedy or controlling by asking about finances and estate planning?
~ Should I move in with a parent? Move the parent in with my family? Or will home modifications keep my loved one independent?
~ Which sibling should be in charge? How can we share duties? What other family members or friends can pitch in occasionally?
~ Does it matter what others think if I have to institutionalize my loved one?

How much help to give, or how little? Assuaging guilt and needing to feel useful can result in giving more attention than is actually needed. Denial, anger, or resentment can result in inadequate caregiving. Overreacting or taking things personally can result in inappropriate solutions. Now it is time to pay attention to how we have built our lives—and what relationship means.

Changing Roles and the Independence Trap

"You would think that in situations like this the family would come together," says John, who cared for his parents for thirteen years, starting at age twenty. "But they don't necessarily, and in my case they didn't; so we had a lot of issues to deal with that were there anyway. Illness can make them better or it can make them worse. If there are any outstanding family issues, it's best to get past them. When everybody is healthy, they have different ways of coping with family members. If you can resolve the issues then, at least you have that part of your life cleared up, which makes it better in dealing with everything else that's coming your way."

Dramatically and unexpectedly, caregiving propels unfinished business to the foreground; not all families rally gracefully. Deciding who should do what can reinvent rivalries or create new bitterness. Says social worker Joan Booty, "Though there are sometimes many siblings, there is usually just one that does the caregiving. The fallout in frustration from other family members can have devastating aftereffects. Parents like to think everyone will come together, but all those competitions from the past come forward, and if these feelings haven't been resolved, it's like being in a pressure cooker."

Experts recommend setting up family meetings that include everyone affected, even grandchildren, and bringing in an objective third-party professional or friend if necessary to ensure that the loved one's wishes are respected but that everyone's concerns are aired. These discussions can be held in person, but meetings can also occur via telephone conferencing, e-mail, and Internet chat rooms for families scattered geographically. Not everything has to be decided at once; short- and long-term agendas can be set and responsibilities divided with one person selected to manage the overall care plan. Nothing is set in stone; decisions can be reversed, even a move to a nursing home.

Although caregiving is often called "role reversal," an adult child never becomes the parent's parent; a wife does not become a husband. Instead, caregiving is about letting go of outmoded patterns to serve the needs at hand. It is a modern twist on the traditional midlife crisis with bountiful clues that we are about to enter a new turning of adulthood. For his book *Once upon a Midlife*, psychiatrist Allan Chinen researched more than five thousand fairy tales—from dreams, anthropology, and mythology—and found "middle tales," stories that shed light on the dilemmas of this phase of life, such as dealing with crises, facing mortality, and honoring the feminine. "Similar dramas appear in middle tales from around the world, suggesting that switching gender roles is a major task for men and women at midlife."

We learn how to be children and we learn how to be adults who take care of children; we learn how to be husband and wife. But we are not taught how to exchange these roles; there are no tidy parameters. To find how to do it, we must revisit childhood and restore the pieces of ourselves left behind while we were busy becoming somebody.

Marty's crisis came in his thirties after his mother had a few episodes of illness that required extensive intervention. Eventually he brought her to California because of digestive tract problems mistreated for years with antacids. Wanting to make her life comfortable after surgery for diverticulitis and knowing that her lifelong Midwestern home had become fouled by gang violence, Marty and his wife, Helena, created a place for Joyce in their new suburban home. They had no clue that the kinetics of growing up as one of five children would reappear twenty years later.

"Was that the biggest mistake I ever made!" laughs Marty, now forty-one, explaining that even though their relationship has softened and deepened, he hadn't lived with his mother since he was eighteen. "There was an undercurrent of unresolved issues that I didn't know existed until we were thrown together and the tables were turned. Instead of her providing the wisdom and support, I was in the position of caregiver, provider of financial help and a roof over her head. Plus I had grown a bit and didn't kow-tow to her thoughts and views on life and politics. She wasn't used to being totally dependent on one of her sons and away from her base of family and friends."

Marty was a child again who felt neither listened to nor part of the family loop created after his father died of a massive coronary when Marty was only nineteen. By nature a positive person, he was game to make a go of caregiving, but old patterns erupted. When Joyce moved in, Marty, a computer salesman, thought he would finally have an opportunity to demystify his father. After she regained a measure of strength, however, every little conversation turned into a confrontation: she saw his questions as an assault on her husband. "That was the flash point in our relationship: from then on, all love and care had to be channeled through my wife so I would not come across as 'Marty not caring.' It was extremely uncomfortable, and trying to bridge that developing chasm became harder and harder."

Marty went into overdrive, trying to be the good son but needing to be his own person. He could not get the recognition that he wanted for his successes. Even though he had been programmed to achieve his dreams, he felt that his mother would bring him down to equalize him with her oldest son, who later died from a crack overdose. Marty worked on defusing his reactions; just when he felt back in control, his wife needed to retire because of depression complicated by the conflicts of caregiving. With tremendous guilt he sent his mother home after nine months, with much discomfort remaining.

Over time, however, they mended their relationship: Marty gave up envying the approval his siblings got and entered a period of high professional achievement. Then he suffered a major medical crisis that kept him out of work for months. During this time Joyce became ill again, with flulike symptoms that turned out to be bladder cancer. She called Marty first, knowing he was the one she could count on.

> Without saying it, she was giving me the respect of being the responsible person I am. I was happy that my mother was able to go into the surgery with positive emotions.
>
> I have found through all this that I love my mother a great deal, but I can stand on my own two feet and be detached because she needs to know that someone has the strength of character to take care of her best interests. If my mom dies tomorrow, she will

go to the grave knowing I was the son she raised. Her passing won't leave me wishing I could have done more. I gave my best.

While it is increasingly acceptable to stay home from work or to miss a social engagement because of a sick child, it is far less so because of an ill parent or spouse. Almost everyone faces these problems at some point, yet almost no one realizes how common they are. One of the subtle factors that complicates caregiving is the "independence" trap: equating maturity and strength of character with going it alone. Dr. Bernie Siegel says in *How to Live between Office Visits*, "If you think that trying to do it all makes you independent, you're wrong. What this does is exhaust you and make you vulnerable to illness. . . . Being independent doesn't mean that you don't need other people in your life. . . . [It] means knowing your ability to deal with adversity as well as expressing feelings, asking for help when appropriate, sharing your needs."

Yet autonomy is at the root of both caregiving and care receiving: it is difficult to ask for help and preserve independence when a person's abilities have declined. Especially for the proud, private generation who grew up during the Depression and fought in World War II, government services can be perceived as a handout, a humiliating end to a life of hard work. The ethos of individualism suggests that everyone has the capability—and responsibility—to take care of oneself. The challenge for families is balancing the decision-making authority that elders need with the assistance required to make sure they're okay. From the perspective of the caregiver, one of the biggest hurdles is getting reliable information on how to be smart consumers of various services.

The Network of Aging Services

It is estimated that a quarter of all North Americans over sixty-five and half of those over eighty-five cannot get through the day without some assistance like bathing or transportation. The Older Americans Act established a web of regional and state offices that coordinate and develop programs for older people, but few people use them until a crisis is at hand and a hospital social worker drops the bomb: find home care, or it's into a nursing home she goes.

Home- and community-based programs vary among cities and rural towns, provinces, and territories; but they include case management, care facilities, respite care, hospice, home health or homemaker services, home-delivered meals, nutrition programs, information and referral, adult day care, transportation, telephone reassurance, friendly visiting, and legal and financial counseling. Many services are free or low-cost, yet most families are out there, floating, until they hit the right combination of medical and social services.

Lack of knowledge about how to manage in a fragmented health care delivery system kicks many families into disarray, as does lack of understanding of physical symptoms. Services must be uncovered and paid for through an overlapping array of providers with different eligibility requirements. An easy solution may become complicated because services are approved based not on need but on funding availability. Because there is no single entry point into the maze of senior service programs—medical, housing, social, legal, and financial problems can all be doorways into caregiving—families may feel pressured to accept the most expedient or the most high-profile option, such as a nursing home, when the actual solution instead may be sound fiscal management, proper hydration and nutrition, or home modifications to accommodate a progressive disability.

For many minority families, the problems of access and availability are compounded by finances: poverty may mean improved access to some services, no access to others. Many minorities lack health insurance and pension benefits, are low income, and suffer from poor health. Most health and insurance programs are developed primarily to serve the mainstream and aren't culturally competent for ethnic minorities. Care providers may restrict access on the basis of citizenship, immigration status, or HMO membership. Minority families may avoid the health care system because of religious beliefs, the pressure of family responsibilities, institutional racism, lack of transportation, lost pay or other employment issues, or ignorance of how to enter the network.

"Access to care isn't always provided to a patient in his or her own language, nor is there respect for or an understanding of a patient's expectations relative to the form of health care provided," says Clayton Fong, executive director of the National Asian Pacific Center on Aging.

Too often, knowledge of services comes too late. "We're like children in a strange and alien world without guidance or direction, and more and more of us are out here," says Faith, whose husband of twenty-seven years died in her arms after a long illness. "Trying desperately to make the right decisions, think the right thoughts, be the perfect caregiver, make our loved one comfortable, happy as possible and feeling as whole as possible in a home not set up for caregiving but for living, entertaining, raising children . . . if only I had had some guidance—how to set up a caregiving room, nutrition and feeding hints, comfort talk."

Yet services abound. The best place to begin looking is your Area Agency on Aging (the local office on aging or senior information and referral). You can also turn to the Yellow Pages under Social Service Organizations and to physicians, mental health professionals, hospital discharge planners, Visiting Nurse Association, local and national medical associations, senior centers, family service agencies, regional offices of Social Security, the American Association of Retired Persons (AARP), the American Red Cross, the YMCA and the YWCA, the Department of Veterans Affairs, and the United Way. In Canada, check with the Division of Aging and Seniors, Health Canada, and federal and provincial services such as the Department of Public Health or Ministry of Health. The point is to begin inquiring as soon as possible and create networks of support along the way.

ACTION STEPS

~ Determine the level and duration of assistance needed at various stages. If your loved one is alert and has only minor physical limitations, requirements may be minimal, such as yard work or running errands. The next level of aid means help in more areas for a loved one who can still live independently. The extreme level of help is when your loved one is cognitively or functionally impaired enough to need continual monitoring, at home or in a facility. Short-term and long-term needs differ, but through poor planning or weak communication, the former can turn into the latter.

~ Watch for warning signs such as a change in attitude or behavior, bills unpaid, the same clothes worn day after day, noticeable weight loss, dizziness, sudden paranoia, and excuses for not going to the barber or doctor. Don't procrastinate if you feel something is wrong. Caring is always an appropriate action.

~ Take your loved one for a geriatric assessment or to a memory disorder clinic at the earliest sign of trouble—if not beforehand.

~ Educate yourself about community resources such as adult day care, volunteers, and home health care, and about the particular condition or disease from which your loved one suffers.

~ Study options for living arrangements, respite care, and professional services such as those provided by an occupational therapist, dietitian, or hospice. Ask questions, even if they seem silly to you. Be persistent—you have a right to information and support, both practical and emotional.

~ Set up a family meeting as soon as possible, including your loved one, to determine options and to create a plan of care. Decide who will be the primary and the secondary caregivers, and be sure everyone has a voice. This is a time to resolve unfinished business and sibling rivalries. Discuss what level of commitment each family member is able and willing to make. Discuss legal and financial matters. Call in a professional if you need someone to mediate.

~ Make a list, with copies to other family members or to professional advisers where appropriate, of personal and financial documents like the following: bank account and credit union names and numbers; safe deposit boxes; will or trust; deeds and titles; stocks, bonds, and properties; insurance policies (names and numbers); birth certificate; Social Security number; credit cards; burial arrangements; important phone numbers, including emergency and neighbors; education and military records; religious affiliation; memberships; lists of employers and dates of service; marriage and divorce certificates; names and addresses of spouse and children; citizenship papers; copy of the most recent income tax return; property tax receipts; mortgage papers; and locations of jewelry and family treasures.

~ Make duplicate sets of keys to the house, car, and boat.

~ Learn the benefits to which your loved one is entitled. These might include disability, health insurance, retirement, family and survivor, Social Security or Supplemental Security Income (SSI), income tax and general relief, and veterans.

~ Be aware of and honest about your limitations in terms of time, finances, impact on employment, and degree of emotional commitment. Delegate responsibility and duties wherever possible. Don't be ashamed to ask for help.

~ Develop networks of support at work and in the community.

~ Verbalize your feelings so that anger and resentment don't build up. There are always options; remain flexible and compassionate. Make time to communicate and listen. Be respectful of what your loved one is going through.

~ Remember that emotional support is always needed on both sides.

Doing the Work Mindfully

Calling their thirteen-year marriage an incredible love affair, Evie and Bill have weathered his progressive multiple sclerosis (MS) with fluidity. "When Bill and I met, he was already having some difficulty," Evie says. "By the time we found out it was MS, we were already madly in love and no way could we stay away from each other. 'Oh, we've got MS,' we said. Neither of us had a clue as to what the future would bring."

Equanimity has been wrought attentively step by step, together. Early on, the couple did a lot of soul-searching and set priorities. On the practical side, they decided to use their modest resources for whatever was needed and to shop smart—the best chair, the best van. On deeper levels, communication is the biggest key, Evie says, and allows them the flexibility to respond to crises with greater openness. Therapy has helped them learn how to let each other know when it is okay to leave Bill alone, for example, so that there are no issues of abandonment or burden.

On the spiritual side, support groups have been an opportunity not just to share concerns but also to learn how to listen. Evie says it's not easy to peel away layers or to address emotions. So she also joined a Jewish Buddhist meditation service at their synagogue, to step back from the reality that reinforces what we cling to in order to find where, as the Tao states, truth waits for eyes unclouded.

The couple has been willing to look at where they are trapped in fear or expectation and to explore the root of suffering together. The dark side is there, Evie says, you can't brush it away; but you can stay with it. Sometimes she wonders if she's in denial because of their joy, yet she knows that she doesn't get so bulldozed by MS's challenges because of solid family support and a belief that caregiving is an opportunity to grow in patience and compassion.

"I always used to say that the purpose in life was to make a difference in the world. But I guess that I make a difference in one person's life—it took a long time to get to that understanding. What is it that we're supposed to be doing? It's right in front of your nose. You don't have to go out there looking."

There is no right or wrong way to do this work; there is just doing it as mindfully as possible. Nor does caregiving end at death: beyond wills and estate sales we are still party to grief, loss, and reflection. When as adults we are asked to take on responsibility for the well-being—even the very life—of someone who is critically or chronically ill, we discover the places within ourselves that are not as secure as we had supposed, not as permanent as we had been taught.

Yet this is what caregiving is: an opportunity to address the concerns about aging, illness, and death that unseat core values. It is a time to redefine our belief systems and priorities. For it is our faith that sees us through when all hope is gone, and it is our courage from which we draw sustenance to do what must be done. It is devotion that causes us to leave the familiar, spirit that guides us home. We begin to learn the value of kindness and to appreciate its power to help us cope. These are the strengths in each of us, and they are called forth when another needs us to come, now.

I Am a Caregiver

Mother's seventieth birthday celebration came a month after the neurologist's confirmation of ALS with a dementia of the Alzheimer's type; Dad had turned sixty-nine two months earlier. I flew home a few days before the party just to enjoy their company. But when I walked into my parents' condominium, I was swamped by regret for having taken them, and life, for granted all these years. Their neat home was filthy, carpets stained on all three floors: Mother was unable to competently carry meals to Dad, who was becoming less and less ambulatory. The fine wood furniture was fogged with dust; there was no hot water, and stove burners were erratic at best. Every twisty and bread tie, every receipt and toothpick obtained over the past several months, every reminder note lay in a lazy Susan on the kitchen countertop. Mother's efforts to hold on to her identity were careening out of control as she began to hoard the refuse of her daily life.

The dishes were clean but my mother was not. The first time I could really smell her was on the way home from the airport, after we repaired to the restaurant bathroom because of her incessant complaining about slipping nylons. Her underthings were the same ones she had been wearing in California, now dingy and safety-pinned together—this from a woman with drawers full of fine lingerie, who had done laundry almost daily and had always dressed immaculately in sensible outfits. Less confident, capable, she had silently curtailed grooming.

My parents refused to be limited by social expectations, medical diagnoses, or fate. They were proudly autonomous, and intended to stay that way. That is what I trusted, anyway, until I watched my father get ready for work the day after Mom almost set herself on fire because she was too weak to light a match properly.

Using a walker to get from bed to sink—showers were now too risky because of instability—Father dressed by leaning on a cane in his walk-in closet. In an elegant three-piece suit and silk tie, on arms steeled through decades of racquetball and golf, he lowered himself onto his knees and crawled to the landing. There he sat and, stair by painful stair, hoisted himself up and then down, panting and grunting for two flights, dragging himself over the landing where he took respite, finally reaching the bottom ten minutes later, crumpled in a heap of frustration and sweat and yelling at my mother who, having wandered off in a haze of distraction, had forgotten to bring his walker so he could proceed to the garage and into the car.

The skein of my life began to unravel, dangling without form or future. So it was that I assumed care of my parents, safeguarding them and keeping them together, to return as best I could the full measure of love they had given me.

I became a caregiver, a term I didn't hear until six months after they had died, in a nursing home, humiliated by fate and unable to salvage lives so well lived.

CHAPTER 2

Women and Caregiving

Kore, the maiden, was picking fragrant flowers in a meadow. She reached for the narcissus, and the earth suddenly opened wide. Out of the depths came a golden chariot drawn by black horses and driven by the faceless Lord of the Underworld. "Mother, Mother," she screamed, "help me!" But Demeter, her mother, was far away.—Tanya Wilkinson, *Persephone Returns*

In legend and folk tale, women typically manifest four roles: wife, mother, daughter, wise crone. In essence they nourish the feminine principles of patience, nurturing, and expansiveness—qualities honed by both men and women through a descent into unknown or long forgotten territory. Mythology teaches that no sentient being is permitted eternal innocence: we all must make the journey into spiritual adulthood to learn the lessons of birth and death and compassion.

Withdrawal from the known world, and eventual reemergence, are well charted in the Greek legend of Kore/Persephone, a maiden kidnapped from the upper world of eternal springtime, then raped and held captive by Hades in the shadow land—what Jungian psychologists call that part of the personality deemed useless and cast into darkness by fears, values, temperament, and cultural bias. Persephone's mother, Demeter, who caused everything to grow, searched every inch of land, wailing for the return of her beautiful daughter. She cursed all fertility in the Earth and in mankind. Everything withered; no child could be born and there was no wheat for bread.

When tumult interrupts real life's comfortable patterns, a person is catapulted into uncharted depths of being. Cherished identities and images are useless in this new land, obscure realms where archetypal goddesses learn to revitalize the neglected parts of themselves before returning to the living with a character tempered by trials. It is a cyclical gestalt—life, death, rebirth—for these feminine roles are not just abstract patterns, but the foundation of all relationship. In storytelling, these principles find depth and luminosity. In sharing, they are beacons to light the way, reminding us of what individuals and society can be.

The Role of Women as Caregivers

Women are traditional handmaidens to birth and also to death: it is most often a female face that a dying person will see. And a needy loved one: More than 80 percent of unpaid caregivers are women. Slightly more caregivers to the elderly are daughters than wives; two-thirds of all caregivers are married and more than half work. Having delayed childbirth, often because of career, more than half are sandwiched in the middle with children under eighteen living at home.

When all these roles are merged, it can seem almost too much to handle—yet women do. Ask Vivian, sixty-six, who has taken on all of these pressures simultaneously—and more than once. Her first daughter died at nine months from cystic fibrosis (CF). Before her third daughter was born, her husband contracted polio. He was in a leg brace and needed some help, but for five years the household was stable. Then her fourth daughter, Suzan, was also born with CF. Vivian recalls:

Suzan required constant care, medication, and postural drainage therapy. It took quite a toll on the family, and although it brought my daughters and me closer, my husband and I grew apart. We were divorced when she was eight.

When Suzan was ten, she became ill and was hospitalized. I took a leave of absence from my job. While I was in Ohio with her, my father, who lived in another state, became ill and died. Suzan became worse and died one week later. I thought my life was over. I was so totally devastated and physically exhausted, and I suppose in shock, that I couldn't take any more. I felt so bad that my father had died alone, and that still haunts me.

Vivian returned to her job—which was lifesaving—and even married the doctor she worked for. "For ten years life was good until he became ill with diabetic neuropathy and was hospitalized for several months. When he was released, I cared for him at home, taking him through the physical therapy. After a year he was walking again. We were blessed." But just when they were ready to retire, her eighty-seven-year-old mother fell and broke her hip. She now lives with them, a situation increasingly difficult to manage. They also worry about Vivian's father-in-law, who is eighty-nine and lives alone.

Yet despite occasional depression and bitterness, she has adapted with a positive outlook. "You have to play the hand that's dealt you, as hard as it may be, and thank God for your blessings. Be glad you can be there for those who need you. My favorite quote is: Live well, laugh often, love much."

If you worry about what might happen, no one would ever take a chance, says Eileen, fifty-two. The baby of her own family, Eileen was always close to her mother. So after fourteen years as a widow, when it came time to choose whom Eleanor would live with, it was not a difficult decision.

At that time, Eileen and her husband had six children at home, aged eighteen months to eighteen years. The family added on a bed and a bath for Eleanor, who had surgery for breast cancer and on her carotid artery. But after Eileen's youngest son started school, Eleanor's memory began to drift, so Eileen quit her job and, eventually, was unable to leave her mother alone at all.

Eleanor became paranoid, thinking her family was stealing from her, especially Eileen's husband. She got upset every time she saw him, behavior Eileen took personally. Eleanor stayed up all night hiding things, then forgot where she had put them. So Eileen stayed up too, spying so she would know where everything was. She became sleep-deprived.

Eventually she couldn't take it anymore, maintaining her own household as well as her mother's finances and house, which Eleanor didn't want to sell. Eileen remembers the breaking point as if it were yesterday: her mother was saying awful things about her and breaking her heart. Eleanor was admitted to a hospital for a two-week geriatric assessment; during that time Eileen realized how hard caregiving had been on her family. At a discharge meeting with doctors and nurses, she was told—in front of her mother—to find a nursing home for Eleanor or risk being hospitalized herself.

Refusing their suggestion, Eileen sought out adult day care, but she was still staying up all night and using a room monitor because her mother had forgotten how to get out of bed and would end up on the floor. Eileen was a wreck, having to be on guard all the time. Her medical problems mushroomed, including gall bladder attacks, high blood pressure, and a hysterectomy. She was trying to be wife, mother, and caregiver: all duties she felt were her responsibility alone.

Keeping the peace made Eileen a prisoner to role expectations. While she was trying to make everyone else happy, she was becoming more unhappy, constantly fretting about relationships. Her children had stopped inviting friends over; her husband had to hide from his mother-in-law's view. The guilt became consuming until she called the local office on aging and the senior center and hired home health aides to help bathe her mother and give her attention. Then she became part of a computer support group, which, with the aid of her family, a local group, and a sense of humor, restored her clarity. Listening to others who had placed their loved ones in nursing homes, she knew the time was coming.

Eileen thought she could never do it, but she did. She and Eleanor discussed it and prayed together about it. On moving day she felt guilty yet also relieved—she slept for the first time in months. But the next day when she walked in, her mother said she hated her and never wanted to see her again. Undaunted, Eileen visited daily for months. Even though Eleanor said she wanted to go home until the day a stroke stole her speech, Eileen was grateful she was able to be a wife and mother again, though she wished things could have been different. Eventually Eleanor passed away at age ninety-three.

> What I have discovered about myself through all of this is that I'm strong and a survivor, and with help I can get through anything. Life isn't always as we want it to be: we have to learn what things we can control and what we can't, and learn to deal with those the best we can. There are so many good people out there willing to give of themselves to others. It isn't a weak person who asks for help; it takes a *strong* person. Loving my mom so much was a key— you love them and you help them when they need it. It was love that kept us all from going crazy.

Women are socialized to nurture connection, says licensed clinical social worker Jeanette Kadesh, a counselor with Jewish Family and Children's Services and caregiver to her own mother for more than twenty years.

> We don't ride off into the sunset; we stay connected to our children and parents. So women end up, because of relationships, being in more of the hands-on role. At the point when most women become caregivers, they are also dealing with their own midlife issues, with children and marriage and work—a lot of tugs and pulls. Caregiving is an especially vulnerable time and a season to acknowledge our own aging processes. There have been years of development where the task is to separate from parents. Midlife is a time when we think we'll be liberated as a woman, but everyone's coming back to the nest.

Women's caregiving is like a baptism into the cycles of nature. In *Women Who Run with the Wolves*, Jungian analyst Clarissa Pinkola-Estés describes the tasks of this journey as represented in the old Russian tale of Vasalisa, who undergoes an initiatory process to develop her intuitive nature.

Restricted by behaviors taught in order to get along in the world, women have imprisoned their natural insight and skills that rescue them when powerless, stuck, or volatile. But there is wisdom in the instinctive psyche, which rises through our crumbling structures. Learning to allow our vitality to be expressed, in letting the "too-good mother" die, our formidable powers of judgment and intuition can blossom. Then roles can be fulfilled from the strength of self-expression rather than inhibited by social pressures. Pinkola-Estés writes: "To be strong does not mean to sprout muscles and flex. It means meeting one's own numinosity without fleeing. . . . It means to be able to learn, to be able to stand what we know. It means to stand and live."

Women and Long-term Care

The problems of old age and long-term care are primarily the problems of women. It is largely a question of numbers: everywhere women outlive men. Longer life comes at a price, however: women are much more apt to be widowed, poor, and without adequate support and resources. Older women are also more likely to be living alone or in nursing homes. They enter old age with more chronic conditions and functional disabilities than men: ravages such as Alzheimer's, osteoporosis, and vision and hearing losses disproportionately affect them.

In all regions and practically all countries, women account for the majority of the older population, a proportion that increases with age. The number of women worldwide aged sixty and over is expected to more than double between now and 2025, with most residing in developing nations. In many countries, more than 50 percent of women over sixty-five and more than 80 percent over eighty-five are widows.

Although the poverty rate among older people has been reduced overall, the number of poor older women has actually increased: nearly three-quarters of the U.S.'s elderly poor are women. According to the Older Women's League, a quarter of all older women live in or near poverty; older women living alone are especially at risk.

Older women are not only more likely than men to need long-term care, they also are more affected by needs of chronically ill family members. Because women tend to marry older men, they are more likely to have spouses in long-term-care facilities. If they haven't done careful estate planning—because they aren't aware of the options or cannot afford the legal fees—many elderly females become impoverished when their husbands are institutionalized because Medicare (a federal health insurance program providing benefits to people sixty-five and older) does not pay for chronic care. Although Medicaid is the largest safety net covering long-term care provided in a nursing home, it comes with a high price tag: in order to become eligible, couples must "spend down" assets to poverty level, often less than $3,000. The amount then allotted to the well spouse at home can leave her destitute, both financially and emotionally.

A third of female caregivers are poor or near-poor, often the "young-old" caring for the "old-old." Child care is expensive, but elder care impoverishes.

The Loss of Work Income

The feminization of poverty among the elderly builds from an early age. More women work in lower paying jobs without pensions or benefits. They take time out of the workforce to care for family members, both children and elders. Often delaying their own medical care because of lack of insurance, many older women are one illness away from welfare.

Although elder care is said to be the newest trend in corporate benefits, it helps only a fraction of working caregivers. Dee found this out when she was thirty-two and her father was only fifty-five. Her caregiving began seven weeks after she had her first son. Her father, who lived with them, began to suffer two to three heart attacks a year, finally succumbing to bone cancer that killed him in six months—at the same time as she was raising three sons and working part time and her husband was starting his own business.

A year after Dee's father died, her mother's ordeal began, first with transient ischemic attacks (TIAs), or ministrokes. Four years ago she fell and broke her hip, which began a series of crises. After a hip replacement, dementia set in, followed by incontinence.

Unfortunately, the corporate world did not see or care about my problems, and after ten years with the firm, I was laid off. I could not put in the "after hours" because I had responsibilities at home. This seemed to matter to them, even though I began my work day one hour or more earlier than I had to.

I look now at my beautiful sons and think they turned into
mature, compassionate men because they were exposed to the tribu-
lations of seeing what family is all about. I didn't have to do all
this, but in my heart, I *had* to do it. Who knows where the strength
comes from? It just seems to be a natural feeling to do what one
has to do. Somehow it all passes and you continue. Life goes on.

Two-thirds of caregivers work, a 50 percent increase in a decade.
Yet because of the demands of at-home care, it is not uncommon for
women to curtail hours, to take early retirement or a leave of absence,
or to quit work altogether. Many women who have cut back on employment fear for their future as well as the present. Says one:

> My mother needed care, so she is living in my home. I am work-
> ing only part-time and not earning enough to pay full-time day
> care and keep up with our household budget. Day care is $900 a
> month, but Medicare/Medicaid won't pay for it. Medicaid will pay
> $4,000 a month if I put her in a nursing home, at taxpayer ex-
> pense. I am hurting my future eligibility for Social Security—with
> family raising and caregiving I do not have enough credits. So I
> have nothing of my own because I am dealing with the present.

Judy is also deeply concerned. At age fifty-four, she cared for her
husband, who was eighty-five. All of the household responsibilities fell
to her, so she had to cut back to part-time work. Robert passed away
after a stroke and pneumonia, and his small pension and Social Security payments have ended. She has had many uninsured expenses for
his care—some of the most costly for household damage he inflicted
while in manic states. "My earnings now will affect my pension later
on; this is the time to be earning the maximum, not working part-
time."

For those in low-paying jobs, the lack of workplace support can be
crippling. Studies show that upper- and middle-class women tend to
be primary care managers for their elderly parents. Even though they
are often physical caregivers, too, they do the setting up, says Dr.
Meredith Minkler, a professor in the School of Public Health at the
University of California, Berkeley. Low-income women tend to be
more hands-on, with daily bathing and feeding, so they're the ones

more likely to have to give up jobs. Chances are their employers don't offer pensions or benefits. "Even the Family Medical Leave Act, which grants up to twelve weeks away from work with a guarantee of return, isn't much consolation. For most caregivers, twelve weeks isn't what we're talking about: it's a long-term commitment. We need policies that speak to the nature of what so many caregivers do."

Although unpaid caregiving represents formidable economic savings to all nations, social custom prescribes that women fulfill this role out of love or duty, without public support. And fully 97 percent of paid long-term caregivers are women. Says Karen Sherr, who works with a labor organization to unionize professional home care workers:

> It is culturally expected to care for a parent in the home, yet it is viewed as "women's work," and we don't value that very much in this society. Society thinks "It's just an old person" and "It's just a woman." Many professional home care workers, most of whom are both women *and* minorities, don't even admit what they do for a living because society holds it in such low esteem, like domestic help or a form of indenture. So there are no benefits—no unemployment insurance, no vacations. It's insulting; and yet this is important work and it keeps people out of institutions, saving the state a lot of money. The social model of health care delivery says that family often give a better quality of care; they should be supported in doing that.

Aging, caregiving, finances, and health are also ethnic women's issues. Minorities are the poorest of poor elderly. Minority older women, especially African Americans and Hispanics, fill the ranks of those who hold jobs without benefits. They are also less well than their white counterparts; their health problems often go unnoticed and untreated. Lack of finances and education are barriers to adequate medical care and disease prevention. African-American women between the ages of forty-five and sixty-four have a disproportionate incidence of heart disease, cancer, and diabetes; they are already at a disadvantage when they become caregivers. And because aging blacks tend to live with their children longer and to have fewer jobs with flexible hours and higher rates of poverty, their caregivers are subject to high rates of hypertension and other illnesses. Yet minority women will become the majority of caregivers in the next century because the fastest growing segment of the elderly is ethnic minorities, who are also the most lacking in health insurance and in need of unpaid family assistance.

Life's Lessons

It can take time to meet major events with open eyes and heart, especially when corralled by laws that ignore the heart. Seventy-one today, with thirty-four of those years in Alcoholics Anonymous, Claudine began her caregiving journey in midlife, when she noticed her husband's judgment was becoming murky. Mike had always been a high achiever, a college graduate and an Air Force officer with a good management position. He had a near-genius IQ, was dignified and handsome, a good husband and father.

But one day in his late forties, Mike came home and announced he had quit his job—too much traveling. He bounced around for five years in low-paying jobs but couldn't hold any of them. His memory got worse and his coordination began to fail. Claudine took him to many doctors; one pronounced it depression and gave him shock treatments. He was basically gone after that, she says. In the Veterans Administration Hospital he was diagnosed with what was then called chronic brain syndrome—before there were diagnostic tools, support groups, or even public awareness of Alzheimer's.

Claudine worked in a high-pressure, well-compensated job in the freight business; her mother, who lived with them, looked after Mike during the day. But other problems surfaced: Claudine's son had a psychotic breakdown; her mother became senile and mean; and her daughter got a divorce and moved back home. Then, as her work became more demanding, Claudine developed ulcerative colitis, resulting in uncontrollable bowel movements. Her doctor said the stress would kill her if she didn't put her husband in a nursing home and get some rest.

Claudine was advised to make a decision that ripped out her heart. Her lawyer, her doctor, and Mike's doctor convinced her to get a divorce—in name only—to keep some assets and a roof over their heads in the event he lived for several years. The fear was that if

Mike went on Medicaid, the state could put a lien against her home and other assets; by divorce, she would be protected. She found a woman who took him into her nursing home for only his Social Security payments. Mike died at age fifty-seven, before Claudine could apply for welfare; she paid every penny of his care, thankful for nerves of steel.

The aftermath, however, was crushing. She was shunned by church members, co-workers, and relatives. The only support came from Mike's family, who knew that in the eyes of God the divorce was her only survival tactic. "Everyone thinks that Medicare, the government, or little elves take care of custodial care. They are the ones who also say, 'What will people think?' and are the same people who are the least likely to help you in any way."

Eventually her mother also was placed in a nursing home, where she died two years after Mike. Claudine had stayed at a job she hated for twenty-five years to have insurance, food, gas, and the wherewithal to keep her family going. She paid a steep toll that will never be recovered: She has had bladder cancer and a femoral bypass, temporal arteritis, polymyalgia rheumatica, and surgeries for two aortic aneurysms. Her blood pressure can get dangerously high despite medication, and she is prone to relapses of polymyalgia. Her doctor says that years of caregiving stress would have killed a less determined person because her immune system had nearly collapsed.

Retiring at age sixty, Claudine drew her pension and her husband's Social Security and sold her big home that had so many bad memories. Then two more aunts required her care; a third is currently in a good nursing home. Today Claudine curls up with a piñon wood fire and books on the pre–Russian Revolution, grateful for her fine solitude. "Looking back, I don't see how I could have done anything differently. I just did what I had to do. I was raised to do what was socially acceptable, to be a caregiver, the solid rock of the home and at all times a lady. What has seen me through is a deep, abiding faith in God's mercy and grace. Stress can kill—but I have learned not to be a martyr or to feel guilty. You don't have to go down the tubes with your loved one."

"Although life is full of unchosen circumstances," writes Jungian analyst Jean Shinoda Bolen in *Goddesses in Everywoman*, "there are always moments of decision, nodal points that decide events or alter character. To be a heroine on her own heroic journey, a woman must begin with the attitude . . . that her choices do matter. . . . She either grows or is diminished by what she does or does not do and by the attitudes she holds."

Attending to illness and death, a woman discovers that perpetually "being nice" in order to get along has alienated herself from her true inner strengths. In addressing her worst fears, in facing life from cradle to grave, she reestablishes the rhythmic process from which great knowing and peace emerge. For there is no life without loss, no birth that is not rebirth. Everything is bound up together.

As long as caregiving is considered women's work, as long as aging and long-term care are topics left on the back burner of policy, the female soul will remain hidden and the deep knowings that connect humankind with its essential nature will remain threatening. Maturation sometimes requires the dying of what we have been in order to evolve. Especially in a world where gender roles are in flux, family caregiving rearranges female identity. The ways women have been socialized to be—submissive, silent, soft, compliant—do not get this job done. Women must struggle to override patterning and reconcile caring with self-care, honoring with letting go.

Caregiving is a time of toughening and learning through phases where we leave "the old parents of the psyche" for a remote land. Yet it is there that we heal the wounds inflicted by agreements we made in our youthful naïveté, when we opted for acceptance rather than wholeness. Letting live and letting die is the natural rhythm women are meant to understand, says Pinkola-Estés: "For most women, to let die is not against their nature, it is only against their training."

Shadow traits that have been denied and buried are now witnessed and allowed expression, softening great emotional charge into more soulful expression. In these tests of endurance and sacrifice, a woman comes into her own. Suffering no fools and becoming master of her new world, she has birthed herself this time from her own dark and fruitful womb.

The Spirit of Christmas Present

When I was a teenager, I couldn't wait to be on my own. At twenty-one I graduated from college and followed my older sister, Marcia, to California. Now those miles had become an albatross: I needed be with my parents, to absorb their love. So when they asked me to come home six weeks after my previous trip to relieve my aunt Sam, who had left her job and home in Oklahoma to look after them, I leapt at the chance. But what I really sought was to rescue them from death.

Sam met me at the airport; Mother was waiting in the car, bundled against the December chill. Her eyes quickly found me. But the sight of her both thrilled and destroyed me: her body had already become thinner, her speech thicker, her eyes less certain. Her weakening spine spelled out a backward "S"; she could no longer hold her head erect.

At home Father was beaming, waiting in his new hospital bed in the living room, vital as ever. I rushed into his arms, and his firm embrace reassured me that he could never leave. All the world fell away as my parents once again became my refuge. Just being in their presence restored my faith: when I was with them, no matter how sorry I was for all of us, I was still safe and they were still alive.

Living with them again, I ached over the changes in their lifestyle. Dad imagined he could be the mind and Mom the legs, but it was not to be. Now a third person would always insinuate into their marriage, taking over the ordinary attentions that fuse a relationship. I was not becoming my parents' parent but their caretaker, friend, and confidante.

Mother was losing ground quickly: a pound a week, countless gray cells. Routine activities were receding even though she would fixate on them, asking about the mail or picking lint off the floor, punctuated by fits of anger or petulance. Her pleasure was going to the piano several times a day to play whatever Rachmaninoff or Bach she still could, making us sing along though we would rather have not. Music was her link to spirit, the essence of her identity, and the only activity still truly her own.

We three developed a full schedule, twenty-hour days filled with meals and hygiene but also errands, picture albums, television, and crossword puzzles. At night, putting Mom to bed took an hour; she could barely negotiate buttons anymore and always wanted to show me her clothes or résumé, vestiges of a hazy pride. When she went to the bathroom, I quickly swept through her nightstand to remove the hoarded lozenges and bits of muffin so there would be no chance of choking. Pillows had to be laid just so; bedspread and sheets smoothed out. I tucked her in with a comic flourish and she'd laugh, then smack her dry lips until they were moist enough to allow her to speak, usually about her long-deceased parents whose framed picture guarded her sleep.

Mom then made sure her eyeglasses, minuscule bits of Kleenex, and her flashlight were at bedside, and when she was certain everything was secure, we kissed goodnight. "Our love will *never* end" was her singsong phrase, always ending with "Thank you for *every*thing." Although it was hard to leave her, I always went downstairs afterward for time alone with Father.

Yet in this journey of love and loss, I learned the meaning of faith the only time I ever celebrated Christmas with my mother. Although I have not been a practicing Jew since my teens, I was raised in Orthodox tradition, the ethics of the Fathers. In high school I was allowed to go caroling if I skipped over the words *Jesus* and *Christ* in every song. My marriage to Bob, Irish and Protestant, tested kinship bonds. Initially my parents renounced our union, but they soon realized that the spirit of the law was more important than its letter. Father was uncomfortable with ritual, but his faith was steeped in ecumenical wisdom and charity. Mother, by contrast, was deeply religious: she consecrated each day to the King of the Universe and at night asked God to bless everyone she knew. Fiercely proud of her Jewish heritage, she nonetheless had grown to appreciate the wisdom of other traditions.

One night Mother led me upstairs well before bedtime. She shut the door and punched on a Luciano Pavarotti Christmas television special, then crawled under her pink afghan and invited me to join her. She sang, we sang the words *Jesus* and *Christ* out loud together, and Mother cried and I cried as she put her head against mine and said she was so very blessed and happy. Although I felt myself slipping down a perilous edge, both joy and sorrow fell with me. Why, I wondered, did it have to take catastrophic illness to teach the meaning of love?

CHAPTER 3

The Medical/ Financial Maze

It is natural, even instinctive to prefer comfort to pain, the familiar to the unknown. But sometimes our instincts are not wise. Life usually offers us far more than our biases and preferences will allow us to have. Beyond comfort lie grace, mystery, and adventure. We may need to let go of our beliefs and ideas about life in order to have life.—Rachel Naomi Remen, *Kitchen Table Wisdom*

Caregiving reposes on three supports: the health care system, finances, and family. It is an uneasy alliance at best: if any part crumbles, they all fall down. The most common gateway into family caregiving is a medical crisis, yet finding the best doctor, the right diagnosis, the perfect rehabilitation plan, and proper financing can be exasperating. Especially in an era of cost-conscious reform, families come up hard against impossible situations: unfamiliar doctors in a hospital emergency room asking whether your spouse should have life-sustaining treatment, a different physician for every medical appointment, training a new home health aide every time one doesn't work out, figuring out how much is owed or what services are covered.

It is all this, and so much more. Families complain that doctors ignore their wishes, that care is not a dialogue, and especially that they are not informed about what a medical diagnosis means over the long term nor are they consulted about treatment. Lay people are expected to understand prognoses, billing and reimbursement, and medication management. There may not be time, or inclination, for a medical professional to discuss fear and grief or the nature of post-surgery home care. Decisions are often made in haste, so families abdicate to experts. When a wife is in shock or a daughter numb with disbelief, she is asked to make the most critical judgments—with clear head and conscience. In crisis, we are expected to be sane; in crisis, we are terrified of killing our loved ones with an ill-informed decision.

"I think modern medicine has become like a prophet offering a life free of pain," writes thanatologist Elisabeth Kübler-Ross in her memoirs. "It is nonsense. The only thing I know that truly heals people is unconditional love." Underestimating the wisdom that lies within, we wait to be listened to, and so, in caregiving, we begin to listen to ourselves. We come to understand that most medical practice can only react *to* us, and to only a part of us. It cannot heal us because it cannot relate to us at our essence. We have sought the quick fix, but it is a lifetime that brings us to this fractured place, and it will take another lifetime to make us whole again.

The Labyrinth of Health Care

A medical emergency confronts families with awkward health care choices that not even professionals always feel equipped to make. To our alarm and frustration, now we understand how much authority has been handed over to people who have less familiarity with and less concern for our dear ones. It is so intimidating: we have given away our power, our hearts, and our wisdom, and when we need them the most, we feel abandoned. We have relied on experts to tell us what to do; even when they respond, we still feel bereft.

Caregiving exposes the underbelly of a medical system that has compartmentalized people into body, mind, and spirit—an abstract mechanism to be probed rather than a dynamic organism to be cared for. Patients want to be listened to rather than dismissed; families want to participate, yet have no background for such a partnership. Both sides are party to health care systems trying to contain costs; both come up against personal and institutional barriers that are difficult to understand and overcome.

The medical maze has other loops: family caregiving disturbs the very foundation upon which we have built our belief systems. It is no longer just physical and financial symptoms that come into play, but our entire perception of life and death. We have been lulled into believing that death is an error because cure is the prime goal of modern medicine. And so we run from treatment to treatment, resigned to a system that pits us against the course of nature until we run dry and discover that what we have been chasing after is not curing but healing: a way to look at illness and death, at nature itself, and find not only acceptance but especially a place in its perpetual rhythms.

Although this century has seen miraculous progress in eradicating infectious disease, as longevity has increased we have also witnessed a surge in chronic illnesses such as heart disease, hypertension, hearing and vision loss, diabetes, and arthritis. Many older people have not just one but several of these conditions. The result is that more families are becoming guardians of long-term care for the medical system, but without proper guidance.

Tom entered this maze years ago while visiting his elderly parents, Pauline and Scotty, three hundred miles away. He found a pile of health care bills, Medicare explanation forms, and collection letters. Though his parents had tried, they couldn't manage the record keeping and were afraid of damaging their credit or, even worse, losing medical coverage. Tom offered to handle the problem but soon slalomed between Medicare and service providers, pressured to pay balances due when he didn't know what was really owed. He became enraged with Medicare and insurance companies that generated so much paperwork without responding to requests for help.

So he plunged into a paper-and-pencil project—which years later he translated into software—to decipher how these payment systems charge for services and how they reimburse. It took him most of a year. Meanwhile, he began to comprehend how his parents' health problems had contributed to their financial woes. Pauline's mental skills had been eroding long before a proper diagnosis, and doctors had been treating her unsuccessfully. Because they were heavy drinkers as well, Pauline reached the point where Scotty could no longer manage her. So she was admitted to a nursing home.

Scotty was adamant about remaining at home, even though he wasn't in any shape for good self-care. Tom became wedged in an impossible quandary: he had to balance Scotty's wish for independence and hopes Pauline would return with his own desire to provide top care. Since Scotty refused to come live with his son's family, Tom wanted him in an assisted-living environment. He agonized over what could happen if he let his father, a heavy smoker, have his way: he could set the house on fire with an unattended cigarette, or while drunk, he could fall and die before anyone discovered him. On the other hand, preserving his father's right to independence seemed more ethical. Was it irresponsible to allow Scotty to live alone? Was it more responsible to place him in an institution against his will?

Tom pursued the best course, finally entrusting the answer to faith. "I decided I had no right to deny his independence in exchange for conditions that would make *me* feel good. With the exception of my wife, Fran, the rest of the world killed me with criticism—family, pastor, doctor, public health authorities. They could criticize till the cows came home, but I was the one who would have to live with the results of my decision."

The next three years were despairing: Tom had to accept that he had no control, and he disciplined himself not to worry. He visited Scotty when he could, making the occasional emergency run with him to the hospital because of dehydration and other problems. Then one night his father said he was ready to accept help. He moved to a care facility and gave up his whiskey and cigarettes. Three weeks later he fell, shattering his hip and undergoing emergency surgery. He told Tom to go home and be with his family; shortly thereafter, Scotty died.

"There is only so much control you can exercise over life," Tom says now at age sixty. "Knowing at the time what is the right thing to do may not be possible. When faced with that condition, look within yourself and find the point that produces inner peace, balancing willingness to accept consequences which won't produce shadows of guilt—and there you'll discover the best thing to do. There is a distinct difference: the right decision is not always the best decision. The right decision would have been to place Pop in assisted living even if it was against his will. The best decision was the one that gave him the happiness he wanted."

Pitting a novice's understanding of medicine and finances against the formal bureaucracy requires tenacity and focus. The bottom line is not monetary but personal. We must be willing to go against the tide if necessary and place spirit at the center of our concerns. "The medical system is just the child of the culture," says psycho-oncologist and author Rachel Naomi Remen. "All of a culture's strengths, dreams, illusions, limitations, and wounds will be reflected in its medical system. The shift in perception, belief, and attitude that will heal our medical system and the people struggling to serve it is the same shift in perception, belief, and attitude that will heal us all."

Financing Long-term Care

"Anyone who says we have the best health care system in the world obviously has never been through caregiving," says John, who cared for both his parents for thirteen years in a climate that made it almost a clandestine activity. "People don't realize the amount of administrative burden on caregivers—the medical, financial, legal problems, all the things that indirectly are going to help the patient but that aren't the hands-on talking, holding, the real *caring* part of caregiving. No one has a concept of the amount of useless paperwork and administrative hurdles you have to jump when you have an ill elderly parent."

Although only 5 percent of those over sixty-five reside in a convalescent home at any one time, health care funding remains high-tech rather than high-touch, skewed toward expensive institutionalization and acute care rather than covering services that would keep families independent. "We have created a health system that is brilliant but irrelevant to the health needs of most older people," says gerontologist Robert Butler, founder and director of the International Longevity Center in New York.

Because virtually no insurance covers all custodial care—standard health care policies pay for less than 1 percent of long-term health care costs—home care can become as costly as institutionalization, especially if the illness is catastrophic or progressive. Many middle-income families become caught between reality and policy, their first contact with the elder care labyrinth both a medical and a family crisis when they discover that Medicare does not reimburse for the bulk of long-term-care needs—and they are left to fend for themselves.

Certified financial planner Tim Millar says that for some people, growing old is like playing the lottery.

> If you get a disease where the treatment is in an acute-care hospital or outpatient [care], then that's covered by Medicare. If you happen to be unlucky enough to get a disease which involves long-term care, then the same programs that protect you for other diseases don't protect you for this one. It should be health concerns that dictate health treatment, not health care policy.
>
> As for long-term-care insurance, if you don't buy a policy when you're young and healthy it can be difficult to obtain at all because the underwriting standards are extremely severe: for example, if you have a parent who has any condition that might result in going into a nursing facility, you will not get coverage. The moral is: this is a much more complicated issue than most people realize, and unfortunately most people realize it when it's too late to do anything about it. If you take action in advance, almost all these issues are solvable. You can't wait until the problem is there.

Older people say it isn't a stroke or dementia that frightens them most; it is being sent to a nursing home. According to Patricia McGinniss, director of the California Advocates for Nursing Home Reform, the lack of financial and respite support is one of the greatest family woes. She bemoans the choices available when a loved one can no longer remain at home, the most heartbreaking decisions made because families fear losing everything as much as being stigmatized as uncaring:

> We do not have affordable, accessible home care for people. The benefits available under Medicare are still very sporadic, the requirements stringent, the care spotty. Under current law you can spend all your savings for in-home care and drive your own health into the ground. Then when the burden becomes too heavy, you

can pay for home health care. There's no public assistance until you spend down to nothing. Although it's not necessary at this point to get a divorce to prevent spousal impoverishment, still the incentive is this: choose between impoverishment and putting your spouse in a nursing home. Everybody knows that people are better off if they can stay at home, but nursing homes are unavoidable for some people and always will be.

These old welfare laws put forth a terrible attitude about the poor—that you did something wrong—and it extends to people in a nursing home. You may not be poor, but if you live long enough in a nursing home, you will end up in a Medicaid program and they will put a claim on your property. They don't tell you this when you apply; rich people get estate planning done. Poor people without disposable income, they don't know that they don't need to lose their home. This is the only so-called civilized country in the world where we think of putting a claim on your home if you happen to be one of the unlucky people who ends up in a nursing home on Medicaid. Nobody should be forced into this position.

Relying on Experts

Because we live in a world where stresses increase exponentially with the light speed of new communications technologies, we look to experts for the quick, definitive answer. But in our busyness we have also become careless. We have let others dictate our needs and values and have ignored our own wisdom. Now we are trapped between distrust of the health care system and lack of connection with inner guidance systems.

We have directed much outrage and bitterness at the medical system, but we have also been smug about our own responsibility for health. Caregiving is instigating a change in habitual response patterns. Families are no longer relying solely on the ivory tower of expertise but are developing their own complementary knowledge. For it is not academic degrees that matter, but the quality of care given.

"Sometimes I think doctors should spend a month or two as a full-time caregiver so that they would have a better understanding," says Dan, who cares for his wife, Doe, diagnosed with multiple sclerosis almost thirty years ago; they are both sixty-five. "Never in my wildest dreams did I think at the age of thirty-seven I would begin a journey as a caregiver and by fifty-seven would be totally responsible for the day-to-day care of my wife. Who would have ever dreamed they would be changing a urinary catheter, suctioning air ways, dressing wounds, and digitally assisting bowel movements in addition to managing food and water intake and keeping records? Who would ever believe I could run a skilled nursing home for one with a staff of one?"

Dissatisfaction runs deep with mechanical medicine that merely prolongs existence. Alice, who had to place her mother in a nursing home after paralysis from several strokes, says:

People were more interested in continuing my mother's life because of what everybody else got. For example, the doctor gave her a CAT scan when she was dying because she had a headache. She had to tell him three times she didn't want to be hooked up to a machine. I got the impression that this is all normal procedure, but nobody complains. There was always the undermining thought that these are professionals, and who am I to say anything—they must know what they're doing. They pushed for one direction and didn't realize how those tests, prolonging life, can be horrible. Naturally you want your parent or loved one to live, so you accept professional advice. You're always being told that this is what's best for the patient. She wanted to end it, but the effort was to keep her going. Everyone was just following a procedure, but they couldn't understand this was a person, not a job.

Bernice and her mother, Ida, lived together all their lives. Ten years ago, Ida became ill with respiratory problems. Over seven years and two especially painful periods, Bernice, born deaf and now sixty, was Ida's sole caregiver. During the first long episode, Ida's regular physician threw tantrums when Bernice insisted on joining her in the examining room. They dumped him. When Ida was hospitalized for congestive heart failure three years later, she was assigned to a physician who disregarded the "Do not give this medication" list and IV'd her for five days, sending her into a tailspin. They changed doctors, and drugs, and Ida improved.

The second and most agonizing stretch was three weeks before Ida's death, after a fall that broke her hip. First, Bernice had to decide if her mother should have replacement surgery at age eighty-eight. It seemed drastic, but the doctor insisted she could handle it, so Bernice agreed. After five days in the hospital, Ida was transferred to a nursing home because, although it was expected, Bernice had become too disabled to care for Ida herself.

One day, Ida had to use the toilet. Bernice asked an aide to come, but she refused. And so her mother was left sitting in her own excrement for over an hour, all the while screaming at her daughter, who watch helplessly. During the third week Bernice and her sister decided they would care for their mother at home, but before they could make arrangements Ida lapsed into a coma during inhalation therapy. She died four hours later.

At the time, Bernice didn't know of anyone who could, or would, have helped out. Ultimately, it was the little moments of touching and holding, cherishing her mother's presence, that saw her through. "If you do the best you can, no one has the right to expect more than that, and you should be proud of what you have accomplished. The best caregivers are those who comfort with their gentle touch, give smiles that are real, pay attention to small details that show they care. We were more than mother and daughter; we were best friends. I could have done no less, but I would have done more if I could."

"Medicine has had such a paternalistic attitude toward patients," says Jean Shinoda Bolen. "It's a hierarchical discipline, and the person at the bottom is the patient. The attitude is that the patient is supposed to be a good soldier, an obedient body that does what she's told." But family caregivers are beginning to discover the power of devotion over that of expertise.

Taking Back Control

"Long before there were surgeons, psychologists, oncologists, and internists, we were there for each other," writes Rachel Naomi Remen in *Kitchen Table Wisdom*. "Becoming expert has turned out to be less important than remembering and trusting the wholeness in myself and everyone else. Expertise cures, but wounded people can best be cured by other wounded people . . . for the healing of suffering is compassion, not expertise."

When caregivers first assume their duties, there is both belief and hope that everything will go smoothly. It is almost a blind faith: nothing really terrible could happen to ones we love. Yet such things do occur. It is not that health care systems are evil, but that most of us are ill-equipped to navigate clearly. But we are not helpless. Caregivers are learning—and teaching others—how to negotiate impersonal medical and financial systems at a time when the most personal attention is needed.

Self-empowerment through mindful involvement is becoming the hallmark of the caregiving experience. Although families rely on the medical profession for skilled care, and gratefully for the most part, they are wresting back control over the most intimate decisions through intense work: gathering information, talking with professionals and other caregivers, planning for the future, and simplifying other aspects of their busy lives. Families are gaining a surprising measure of competence that enhances professional input. With as much territory covered as possible, caregiving becomes teamwork rather than an island of frustration and anger. Taking responsibility has another benefit as well: it leads to self-knowledge, exposing the faces of the soul.

Stan is a retired certified financial planner in his sixties, a tax expert with a real estate license. He is financially comfortable, with four children who remain close. Nothing, however, including wartime naval service, prepared him for caring for Irene, his wife of forty years.

If you survive several years of full-time primary care, you are changed forever. You find out who you are in this demanding thirty-six-hour-day equivalent. You find that you have a "helpless human being" who is totally dependent on what you do or don't do, and if she were all alone, she would not survive more than a few days. So you work with what you know, quickly learn what you do not know. Then you decide whether you pay someone else or learn and go on. You have to learn to take care of the care receiver.

The traditional father, Stan was unprepared for running a home. But today he fixes meals, and his floor-washing and -waxing skills are superb. Home cleaning, shopping, running errands, and grocery planning are in his proud arsenal. He uses his financial background to reduce their burdens: if Irene spent ten years in a top nursing home, the outlay would approach a million dollars. With legal fees running $200 an hour, he quickly learned to do the preliminary homework— prepaid funeral planning, estate planning, wills, codicils, living trusts, and end-of-life planning such as tube feeding and "Do Not Resuscitate" decisions.

Stan says that relying solely on doctors for information about Alzheimer's is inadequate and a prelude to disaster. To assure that Irene will be properly cared for, Stan has devised an adjunct curriculum: studying the immune system, nutrition, and blood pressure, and learning which medical specialty does what. He subscribes to newsletters and accumulates medical books and encyclopedias on drugs. Long-term planning has meant choosing doctors, neurologists, medication, and hospitals and evaluating day care centers and nursing homes. The sweep of his decisions must cover his own survival until Irene's death, then the remainder of his life as well as contingency plans should he predecease her.

On a physical level Stan has learned how to change Irene's diapers, feed and bathe her, and move her around with a cast on her leg after a fall. He has done all this despite his own battles with high blood pressure and a fall that cracked two ribs. It wasn't so long ago that he was nearing breakdown. Although Stan began each day feeling fine, at the end he would feel like a rubber band "stretched to the limit and ready to snap in two or rebound all over the place." Today he religiously takes short breaks or plays at the computer to release tension. Physical fitness is also part of his regeneration: having given up running after logging twelve hundred miles a year, he is now back in full force, planning participation in marathons in London and a few global odysseys.

He regained his fortitude after a strenuous Alpine climbing trip, his first true respite in years. He returned with a new spirit to handle his commitment and discovered that Irene could manage in his absence. Having faced the big questions of life and death, having been mightily tested, he has developed not just skills but also perspective.

I know who I am now—I'm stronger, smarter, and a real survivor, able to handle any situation. This only comes when the chips are down, you are in a crisis mode, and you acquit yourself well. The pain of the adult caregiver can be lessened by recognizing that life is not fair . . . and never will be. If you provide loving care and then can go on to life on your own, you are a new person. You accept that everyone dies eventually; life is precious. You achieve a great inner feeling of joy and satisfaction that comes from caring for your special one.

ACTION STEPS

~ Obtain a booklet about Medicare and Medicaid coverage from your local Social Security or health insurance counseling office. Study it carefully to be an informed consumer, especially ahead of a crisis.

~ Obtain a personal earnings and benefit estimate statement from the Social Security Administration for all potential caregivers and care receivers.

~ Determine your loved one's current and future assets: income, expenses, and debts. Set up a bookkeeping system if there isn't a good one in place. Set up joint financial accounts in case you will need to take over bill paying and deposits. Make short- and long-term financial plans where possible.

~ Find out where your loved one keeps his or her financial and legal papers, and make sure they are current. Consult a certified financial planner and/or elder-law attorney where necessary.

~ Consider the cost of long-distance assistance on your own pocketbook. Review your financial situation for the long term.

~ Obtain a durable power of attorney for health care and for finances and a living will for each care receiver. Consult an elder-law attorney or legal aid adviser about estate planning, guardianship or conservatorship, and living trusts or wills where appropriate. Every step you take in advance frees your time for caring rather than paperwork.

~ Investigate long-term-care insurance and other supplemental health insurance with qualified professionals, including the hospital discharge planner. Check telephone directory blue pages to locate Government Insurance Assistance.

~ Speak to medical professionals, and demand answers if you are dissatisfied with treatment. You have a right to responsible care.

~ Involve your loved one whenever possible in planning and decision making.

~ Call your local Area Agency on Aging or senior information and referral to learn of low-cost or free financial and legal counseling. Don't settle for less than what you need in terms of information and support. These services are for you and your loved one.

The modern health care system is composed of professionals who are as much a part of the web of cultural beliefs as the lay people they serve. In most developed nations those beliefs deny nature and push for extending life, too often at the expense of dignity or desire. We are coconspirators in this interpretation of death as an outrage, absolving our part in it by giving over our power to designated authorities.

"To medicine's absorption with The Riddle [of disease], we also owe our disappointment when we cherish expectations of doctors that they cannot fulfill and perhaps should not be asked to fulfill," writes surgeon and author Sherwin Nuland. "The Riddle is the doctor's lodestone as an applied scientist; it is his albatross as a humane caregiver."

Before he passed away from cancer, Joseph Cardinal Bernardin, archbishop of Chicago, addressed a conference of the American Medical Association. He told physicians that "the age-old covenant—the moral center of the doctor-patient relationship—has been ignored or violated" and is in danger of being lost irrevocably by giving in to financial success, scientific triumph, and political power. Calling medicine commercial and soulless, he said that sustaining physician's covenants requires "a willingness to affirm and incorporate in their lives the ancient virtues of benevolence, compassion, competence, intellectual honesty, humility, and suspension of self-interest."

For hundreds of years, the physician's authority, and perhaps even some of his healing power, has derived from the patient's faith that he can make things right. But healing is only one of the hopes that a patient focuses on a physician, says neurologist and author David Simon in *The Wisdom of Healing*. For many people, particularly isolated elders, a doctor may be the only person who offers a caring relationship. Although precise diagnosis, rather than comfort and compassion at bedside, has become the modern way, illness brings up a cluster of emotional triggers. So there is much that a doctor can bring to the table besides the possibility of getting well. Simon urges that the spiritual practice of medicine keep pace with surgical and medical technologies so that the soul receives care to match that provided for the body.

To heal others we must, as the saying goes, heal ourselves. Just as health professionals must distinguish between technology and nurturing, blending them in a humanistic rather than an emotionally removed partnership, good caregiving derives not out of anger and resentment at impersonal or arrogant medicine, but out of taking responsibility for the tasks at hand. If it means that we must do homework to educate ourselves, so be it. If it means that we must make dozens of phone calls to service providers to make sure we have not been overcharged, then that is the work before us today.

Dealing with medical and financial issues brings us to a difficult place where we must make an investment of time and energy and concern far greater than what we signed on for. This commitment leads not only to better care for our loved one, but also to deep satisfaction and personal growth—and, ultimately, preparation for what is to come. That is no small feat, and one of which we would do well to be mindful.

A Sacred Sorrow

Pilloried by social convention about how women should act, I was consumed by my failure to be superhuman. I appeared pathologically obsessed with grief as I vacillated between childhood and adulthood. Deep waves washed against the shore of my being, pulling me out toward a foreign and terrifying land. Something had hooked me and was leading me I knew not where.

Dad's sister, Aunt Sam, stayed on in Wichita. Profoundly capable, having been a successful retail manager, she oversaw finances and arranged community services such as Meals on Wheels. Reluctantly, Dad hired some help so that Sam could take breaks. Clara, a seasoned home health aide, would do light housekeeping and bathe Mother for about $90 a week, a cost that frightened Dad because there was no financial cushion. He thought they had enough money to last a year if nothing changed; he hadn't counted on needing help. Even though he didn't want their illnesses to become our lives, he vowed he would never sacrifice Mother to his desire for independence. I wanted to believe him.

We all hoped—pretended, probably—that this was as far as their decline would go. But one day Mother was rushed to the hospital; increasingly misshapen and unstable, she had fallen. A hospital social worker was sent to inspect the house and called me at work without warning. She pronounced the condo unfit for my mother because of the stairs. There were some home modifications we could do—extending the handrails at each landing so Mother could reach them from the first steps, putting levers on light switches and door handles—but it wasn't enough. She was refusing personal care (bathing in particular) and risked losing Medicare benefits.

"No one is facing reality," the professional told me. Furthermore, because of the unsafe conditions, the home health agency could face legal problems. She also threatened to call Adult Protective Services, which meant the state would step in, perhaps forcing my parents into an institution. "This much care needed in the home is unusual. When it gets to this level, people are admitted to a nursing home." Impossible, I said; we can't separate my parents. She suggested I remove them together. I buried the matter.

Mother began yelling at Clara in a weak but bossy manner not to take the laundry upstairs or make lunches. She was afraid she would steal something and was reluctant to give up more household roles. Even though Clara knew it was the disease, she threatened to quit almost weekly. Meanwhile my aunt, who suffered from high blood pressure and depression, soon surprised us with the announcement that she would be present only in short chunks of time. Dad didn't understand; he assumed his sister would worry less if she lived with them. He thought she could always get out and enjoy herself. But there was nothing to enjoy in this world: Sam could not bear to watch her brother diminish nor abide her sister-in-law's mutation. I had no clue what to do next.

Despair reached into my being, extended back to my birth, and traversed all the wounds in between, gathering them up and ferrying them to the farthest reaches, branding my soul until I released them into nothingness. "I wish it weren't so," I told my mother in that other-world place. "But it is," she answered back. I had only the power to care for them, not to save them. And so we continued to be whirled away together, to follow this sacred sorrow wherever it might lead.

CHAPTER 4

Caring for Aging Parents

The ways of power ask a great deal of us. When these ways are new to us, it is even more difficult. I wish I could reach into your heart and make you see how important this work is.—Lynn V. Andrews, *The Woman of Wyrrd*

"We remain fixated to the unexorcised images of our infancy, and hence disinclined to the necessary passages of our adulthood," wrote mythologist Joseph Campbell in *The Hero with a Thousand Faces*. When we are young, the universe is inexhaustible, perpetually life-giving and indestructible. No matter how mature we fancy ourselves to be, we are never ready to part with childhood.

Most people who reach fifty have at least one living parent. Because of greater longevity, many adults can expect to care for a parent as long as or longer than their own children—eighteen versus seventeen years. Consequently, for the first time the average married couple has more parents than children. How do we make life-and-death decisions for people who gave *us* birth and who want to remain independent? We are not prepared to see our parents change—the memory lapses and increasing frailty. We come to understand that there are no safety nets, neither in the medical system nor in society.

"Not everyone grew up in a happy family, and suddenly their whole lives revolve around this caregiving situation," says support group leader Cilla Raughley. Here it begins, the end of what was complacent; yet even if we do not know what is to come, we can accept the challenge of giving back, in whatever measure possible, to those who raised us, no matter how we perceive those efforts to have been.

This is my mother and this is my father, and we have been commanded to honor them. Now, in caring for them, we will find out exactly what that ancient devotion comes to mean.

Becoming Responsible for a Parent's Well-being

"This last month has really been hell, no one but me to make every decision," says Maurene, fifty-six, who gave up sixteen years as a Wall Street analyst to move back to London to be with her dying mother. "The responsibility of taking care of her is enormous. It still scares me. I don't feel equipped in any way to deal with this. I seem to hurtle from one 'terror' to the next."

Caring for an aging or ill parent is something none of us expects to do—we associate *life* with our parents. But suddenly we are there, taking care of the ones who diapered us and shunted us to school and sports; here we are now, diapering and transporting them to doctors' appointments. It doesn't seem right and it doesn't seem fair; it seems impossible. Whether we got along or not, the shock of being responsible for the welfare of a parent is unsettling. Says Pat Sussman, implementation director of a social health maintenance organization, "We don't want to think about our parents getting old and dying because then there's nothing between us and death. We're next. And we don't want to look at the psycho-emotional implications."

Family dynamics are different now. Adult children must find ways to help their parents remain comfortable. They must determine when and how far to step in, for how long, and at what cost. They must find ways to bring up uncomfortable topics—legal and financial matters, asset management, housing preferences, end-of-life treatments—without robbing their parents of the power to make decisions. They must recognize old wounds and work through them, dealing with lifelong patterns of behavior and communication—even alcoholism or abuse—that can promote or frustrate this shift in roles. Nothing fits the way it did: our mantle is larger, and we must grow into it.

For Lynn, fifty-one and executive director of a child care consortium, the end of the familiar sideswiped her when, in a two-week period, her mother-in-law, Hilda, showed signs of disorientation and her own mother, Marion, had intestinal surgery. Despite wonderful family support, Lynn, who has four children in their twenties, at times found the transition to caregiver difficult, especially balancing competing demands. With her younger sister, Barbara, who has a toddler and a key position with the consortium as well, they remained devoted to providing the best care possible but were always stretched between family and work. One event seemed to precipitate another: Marion broke her hip and needed surgery, then developed lung cancer and emphysema. After a vibrant life and an enormous farewell party attended by friends and family from all over the country, she decided to save the money being spent on home care and move to a nursing facility, where she passed away five days later surrounded by devoted family. Meanwhile, Hilda is living out her days in a convalescent home, stricken with dementia so advanced she is no longer able to enjoy her children and grandchildren.

"It happens so suddenly," Lynn says. "Your parents are fine one day and the next day they're not, and you're thrust into this whole other world. When I had to worry about my mother, that was a major change. I liked it better when we were young, our children were young, and our parents were young, and I didn't have to worry about my parents. But you can't make people young again. You can't make people happy."

It is not as important that we are daughters or sons or parents but people in new, caring relationships. Parents are at the mercy of their caregivers, knowing in their hearts that they are burdening their children and throwing their lives off course. Adult children are ill at ease and confused, scared because of the implications of long-term illness. They must address these alien emotions while finding practical solutions to the problems at hand, learning to give graciously so that parents don't sense possible resentment or hostility. Research is inconclusive, but one study reported that getting support from an adult child is beneficial at moderate levels but psychologically harmful at high levels. Yet parents who didn't expect much support and then got it cited higher levels of well-being.

Once crisis hits, it is more difficult to find solid footing. We can gain definite advantage by educating ourselves ahead of time about community resources, financial and legal issues, and health and fitness in the elderly. We can address warning signs such as poor hygiene or eating habits, difficulty walking, or being suddenly aggressive or argumentative. Even so, nothing can truly prepare us for the emotional challenges: if we are not in denial, we must plunge ahead.

Caring at Home

In surveys, older people insist it is at home where they wish to grow old—to age in place. But when they can no longer live on their own, often they live again with their children. If it is a long-distance relocation, moving can mean giving up a lifetime of friends and familiar activities, a traumatic life change. But even when it's the adult child who moves back home, there can be significant ground to cover before realizing the richness of family ties.

Rich knows the journey well; it swallowed him up a decade ago, spewing him headlong into troubles he never imagined. During the Loma Prieta earthquake that shook the San Francisco Bay Area, he lost his house. But that loss was nothing compared to what lay in store. Planning to rebuild, he moved into his mother's home thirty miles south, near the college where he is a professor of Spanish. He thought that even if it took a year to recover, at least he would have a roof over his head.

Although over the years he had regularly visited his mother, Lillian, once he moved in, that's when he saw something was terribly wrong. "Mom weighed sixty-nine pounds. She had always kept an orderly house, but every bit of food was rotten or had weevils in it. There were mice droppings all over the place, and her little dog was messing everywhere. She appeared to be living on two-pound bags of M&Ms and as many as thirty-six cups of coffee a day. And she smoked two to three packs of old-fashioned Lucky Strikes every day. It was unbelievable."

At first, Rich thought that Lillian was lonely, her illogical behavior some sort of "little old lady thing." But problems soon multiplied: wanting to help clean up after dinner, she would throw silverware in the garbage can or flush the cloth napkins down the toilet. Her questions became incessant and irritating as she slipped further from being the mother he had always loved.

Rich, then forty-three, kept thinking this couldn't be happening. He and his partner, Robert, started from scratch, throwing out food and cleaning the house. Rich also took over paying the bills. One day his mother accused him of stealing her money and hiding her cigarettes. "I said, 'That's it, I have never stolen anything in my life, I will not be responsible any longer for this.' I went out and bought twelve cartons of Lucky Strikes, threw them on her bed, and said, 'Put them anywhere you want, and don't ever ask me for a pack of cigarettes again!' I know that was childish, but I was losing my mind."

The first step was the hardest, for it meant admitting they needed help. Lillian was given a geriatric medical assessment at the local Veterans Administration Hospital. Rich says, "If you think this behavior is directed at you, that you did something wrong that you don't understand and now why is this person—or worse yet, why is God—doing this to you . . . it's easier to fight the monster if the monster has a name. It was an epiphany. I had never even *heard* of Alzheimer's."

A hospital social worker put them in touch with several community agencies. They hired a home health aide, discovered adult day care, and found resources and companionship in caregiver support groups at a nearby hospital's senior services program. Although they were beginning to get a handle on their situation, the journey was far from over. Rich developed high blood pressure and put on weight; Robert suffered from shingles. They worried they would explode from the cumulative anxieties. In cycles they went through denial, anger, resignation, then begrudging acceptance that nothing about the process was rational or certain. Nothing on this path fit social expectations. Even with some plateaus, caregiving meant waves of decline. Lillian's repetitive and paranoid behavior kept them up night after night; she wanted to go home when she already *was* home. They worried about insulting her dignity by seemingly taking away her independence; they fought with each other and with her.

Then Lillian fell and fractured her hip, which required surgery and then rehabilitation in a nursing home. When Medicare ended coverage after only nine days of convalescence, the pair became frantic over not having enough funds for the rest of her care there. They may have felt like giving up, but they did not. Little by little they realized there was a way through: with a shift in perspective, with continual self-reminders about love and patience, they slowly regained their lives. Robert says: "There's only one thing you can do to alleviate your problem: just love your patient. Don't say, 'What has God done to me?' You must say, 'What has God *given* me?' It may be a tremendous opportunity to learn what real love is, to give all the love that you can give, and become a better human being."

We live by heart and by hearth. Although living with an ill parent is by no means feasible or advisable for everyone—there are other family members to consider as well as finances, space, privacy, lifestyle differences, and unresolved issues—it is a chance not so much to change roles but to deepen them. There is no shame in not being able to live together: we broke off into our own worlds, and others depend on us to maintain them. What matters is to give dignity and attention to a parent's final years, even if that means unsettling our lives, giving up for a time some of our adult dreams.

Generosity restores far more than the accolades or paychecks we may have missed. And it teaches our children the continuity of love.

Extending Families

There are more options today for keeping a parent autonomous than at any previous time. Home- and community-based groups offer a range of programs including homemaker and other "custodial" services in which aides provide personal care such as bathing and dressing or do laundry and house cleaning; and home health care, or medical-based services, including skilled nurses who regularly monitor vital signs. Other supportive aid includes home-delivered meals, senior companions, respite, and escort services. Although they are not generally covered by insurance, these services can make the difference between keeping a parent at home and institutionalization. They ease our continuing commitment; they also make it possible to combine households when an elder can no longer live alone.

According to the Older Women's League, one in five caregivers has a parent living in his or her home. Although it may not always be the best course of action, sometimes it is the only acceptable one. Despite good motivations, unexpected tensions can arise. There is confusion, stress, and a mix of needs and beliefs as we re-form extended families without the traditional stay-at-home mom. But in so doing, we may also find ways to open our hearts.

Twenty percent of caregivers to the elderly are not spouses or daughters but other relatives, such as daughters-in-law. It is an act of filial devotion beyond blood ties.

Forty-four-year-old Edyth Ann is dedicated to her seventy-year-old mother-in-law, Milly, for whom she has been caring at home—not as an invalid but as a full family member—for six years. Edyth Ann felt competent to take on the duties because she had worked in convalescent care and private duty nursing—actually preferring Alzheimer's patients. Although she knew what to expect, it didn't necessarily make the agreement easier.

First, there were relationship problems to overcome. Edyth Ann's husband, Marcus, felt his mother had not been affectionate; Edyth Ann and Milly had merely tolerated each other. There were other family difficulties as well, including trust issues between the couple and a daughter with attention deficit disorder. But once Edyth Ann discovered how much help Milly needed, and how confused and frightened she was living alone, she confronted Marcus with the need to take care of her. Then Adult Protective Services called and asked Edyth Ann to take on guardianship. It was the splash of reality Marcus needed to take charge. They moved into Milly's home, which initially made Edyth Ann feel like an outsider. She closed her grooming shop and became a full-time wife and stay-at-home mother. It was not an easy transition.

"When we are first confronted with something as terrible as the loved one's 'condition,' the biggest emotion is fear of the unknown. Learning about her condition is one of the best defenses." And what an education it has been. Edyth Ann surprised herself: she accepted the diagnosis, discussed possible treatment with the doctor, and devised an appropriate care plan. And as she has trained her family about the stages of the disease—what to expect, how to ease the transitions— she has learned a lot about Milly and even more about herself. The experience has rebuilt the family and repaired the relationship between mother and son.

There have been lows, however, including times the children resented the attention given to their grandmother. It is difficult for the couple to attend their kids' important events together. Outings have been curtailed because someone always needs to be with Milly; and hired sitters are expensive. The family has run a gauntlet of emotions, including anger, resentment, guilt, denial, and fear for the future. Odds are better than 50 percent that Marcus will develop the disease—both of Milly's parents and one of her sisters has it. And what of the children's odds?

Yet the benefits of this arrangement have been undeniable. Edyth Ann says:

Caregiving allows me to openly give love and face my emotions without fear. It has built me into a stronger person, free from worrying about being hurt or judged. It is by denying yourself the right to be human and to have those emotions that they will grow out of proportion. You cannot control what is happening, but you can lend emotional support. Touch becomes important. The ability to bond to someone is important. The desire to feel loved and needed is very important. Now Milly and I have no shortage of love for each other, and my kids move around with her as if everything is normal and as it always has been.

One of the greatest benefits is developing relationships and giving up old ways of controlling. Accepting another person's reality works with all people in my life. I used to try to change my family to make them more of what I thought they should be. This caused great stress and a huge feeling of failure. The best way to change someone's behavior is to change my reaction to it.

Sometimes I get "caregiver dementia," usually after a series of hard days when I am stressed to the max. Nothing to worry about—it is a warning sign that I need time out, some food, and rest. I do juggle my time, but if I omit myself from that juggling, then I am doing them all a disservice. I cook, I clean, I manage household money, I run errands, I wipe the tears—including my own. I encourage others, I strive to grow, I plan and then replan, I give hugs, I wash the clothes and dirty bed linen, I tutor my kids.

We never know what is involved, where our strengths and weaknesses are until we try. Every time I hear "No one cares," I become upset because it just isn't true. People *do* still care, but as a society we have forgotten how and/or become afraid of caring. It is important that we start learning again. Caregiving has taught me that we are responsible to, not for, each other and that relationships are not disposable. It has allowed me to grow in ways that, without it, I don't think I would have grown—I have even fallen in love with my husband all over again. It has strengthened us and bonded us in love.

Placing a Parent

Today there are options other than living with a parent or placing him or her in a nursing home. The fastest-growing among them is assisted living, adult housing that mixes independent units with a range of personal support services. Many facilities are homelike in atmosphere, with few residents; others are larger, with many activities and a range of lifestyles. They are a midway point between independence and convalescence—to fill the gaps when the family cannot. Although they may not be ideal, they can be a salvation.

"Your stepmother is dead, and we think your father has Alzheimer's disease. You need to come home at once." That is how Margaret, a media specialist, entered the arena of long-distance caregiving. An only child deeply devoted to her eighty-one-year-old father, Margaret dearly wanted to be able to take him in permanently or to quit her job in Washington, D.C., and move to Ohio to care for him. Neither option was workable: he lives in a high-unemployment city where good jobs are scarce. The family couldn't afford the $14-an-hour round-the-clock custodial care that he needed—Medicare wouldn't cover it—and there was no one else available to do all the jobs the home health agency wouldn't cover. Historically, in such crises, Margaret says, African-American families have pulled together, making arrangements for an ill elder to live with a relative. But times are changing.

Margaret, forty-seven, took care of her father for a brief stint but couldn't continue. She developed high blood pressure, worn out from staying up nights listening for signs he was wandering out of the house. "I felt so helpless. I didn't know how to watch him twenty-four hours a day. I couldn't see myself changing diapers and feeding and toileting an adult, especially since I would be going through so much emotional pain. I didn't want to have to watch him die by degrees on a daily basis."

She agonized over placing him in assisted living, even though she researched facilities carefully with relatives, who have been close and supportive. She worried whether he would have enough activities and attention and be safe from wandering. Although initially Margaret felt awful, her father is adjusting, and his friends and relatives see him regularly. Even though she calls frequently and visits as often as she can, guilt still hangs over her: there was no other way, even though it was not what her father wanted. She can be pulled off balance hearing that other caregivers have maintained their parents at home. Does that mean she loves her father less? she wonders.

Despite the trauma, Margaret and her father have become closer, appreciating little things with a youthful innocence. One warm day in February, they took a walk in a park near a pond. Margaret recalls, "As we sat on the bench, Dad sighed, looked up at the sky, and said, 'Nature. There's nothing like it.' I don't think we'd shared something like that since I was little. It shouldn't have taken a debilitating disease to make that happen. But I have learned that I can do only so much to make him happy and comfortable because the disease won't allow either happiness or comfort."

In caregiving, we must come to accept the direction life has taken if we are to do our best. It is important to keep all options open, to never say never, for we cannot know where fate will take us and what decisions will be required. Over distance, it is hard not only to plan for care but also to monitor it, especially without help. In some ways, distance also makes it harder to let go because we never had a tight grasp. But even these emotions are manageable in time, for it is a caring heart that sees us through.

ACTION STEPS

~ Involve your parent in as many aspects of planning as possible. Listen to, respect, and have compassion for his or her desire for autonomy and control. Work together to set up a flexible care plan and remember that it can be changed when needs dictate.

~ Monitor or curtail a parent's activities that pose safety risks, such as cooking, driving, or operating machinery.

~ Monitor whether your parent is eating and exercising properly, getting enough liquids (hydration is important for peak mental and physical functioning), maintaining social contacts, negotiating stairs safely, and dealing with other housing elements competently. Assess housing features that may need modification.

~ Work out unfinished business and old wounds—with parents and siblings alike—so that there will be no regrets or guilt about what might have been.

~ Find out where legal and financial documents are kept and who the professionals and advisers are (legal, financial, medical). Assess finances, both yours and your parents', so that if a crisis hits, you have some idea of what options are possible.

~ Educate yourself about resources in your parent's community; talk to professionals early on to learn what options, such as housing and in-home support, are available. Sometimes there are waiting lists, especially for the better nursing facilities or retirement communities; you may want to put your parent on those lists as a precaution.

~ If your parent is uncommunicative, consult a legal or financial professional on your own to learn your options. Bring in a professional or an objective third party if family strains prevent calm, rational discussions.

~ Bring in a professional, such as a care manager, when possible so that you don't feel burdened or martyred. Stay in touch with a parent's physicians.

~ Find a support group, whether at work, through a local hospital, or on the Internet. Even listening can be enlightening and comforting.

~ Use the Internet to educate yourself about a particular condition or disease, and network with professionals and other caregivers on-line.

~ Discuss possible living arrangements before a crisis hits. Be realistic about what it would take to live again with your parent, in his or her house or in yours. What society may tell you is proper may not be the best situation in your particular case.

~ Discuss end-of-life issues and preferences, when possible, to mitigate surprises and to be able to honor your loved one's wishes smoothly.

~ If you live long distance, call regularly. Set up a network of neighbors, family, and/or professionals to monitor your parent and report to you.

Soul Keeping

It can be necessary to uproot a parent, not just for physical well-being but for preservation of their very spirit. For it is not just a body that we are asked to care for: the unspoken role of every caregiver is guardian of the soul, and this prospect can be the most frightening. For where does well-being come but from within? Where does the giving come but from compassion? We are asked not only to be gatekeepers but especially soul keepers, preserving the best in our parents and inheriting the wisdom of their experience. When we are shepherding their lives, we had best be mindful of their spirits as well.

Six years ago Kara, a fifty-four-year-old psychologist, became a caregiver for her eighty-seven-year-old father, who is Native American. She had to bring him to California from his home in the Midwest, where he had retired from teaching and wished to live out his days, close to nature, family, and friends. But through a series of unfortunate incidents after suffering partial memory loss from a leaky gas valve in his apartment, he was judged mentally incompetent. Because of mandatory reporting, Adult Protective Services gave over his care to an agency—which then tossed him out of his home, removed his belongings, and took over his financial accounts.

"In probate court, when they asked how he felt, he did a dance. He tried to tell them he could sing, dance, laugh, and love his family and friends—that was an expression of his culture and spirit," Kara says. "But a judge who had never met my father thought he was crazy, said he could no longer make any decisions about his life, and assigned him to a guardianship agency of strangers."

The only way Kara could restore her father's freedom was to get a court order allowing him to visit relatives in another state. She removed him permanently because he faces institutionalization if he returns. "The issue for me is protecting his freedom and not having his life taken over by people who don't know him. It isn't common sense to protect a person by removing their whole lifestyle. When someone has dementia or memory loss and already has some difficulty in self-expression, he is hesitant to communicate. If you place on top of that a cultural difference, there is added prejudice in terms of not believing that person is still there as a human being."

Kara is adamant about the need for clarification of what constitutes mental competency, as the definition differs among jurisdictions.

As long as he remains away from his home, he is free to make personal choices. The dilemma is, how do you protect a person without removing their rights? You want to give care and protect their spirit, but how do you do that in a culture that separates the person into physical, mental, emotional, spiritual categories? A person's right is not just to live in their own home but to honor their choices. My father is a person whose spirit is still there. There is the issue of safety, but there are other ways to approach this and not ignore the inner life, which should have equal protection.

Caregiving is "the other midlife crisis," says social worker Joan Booty. "It forces you to look at your life and self. Sometimes families who have had a lot of problems are forced to do some introspection when trying to work together with parents. It can be an opportunity to change and come to some closure. It can be a real wake-up call."

When we become caregiver to a parent, we must revisit childhood, mindfully and respectfully, to come into mature understanding of what relationship means, what family involves. How do we perceive and interpret all that went before? How do we bring forward the willingness and the strength to make room for the unknown and the inconvenient, to step in where help may not be wanted or where we have not felt well parented?

The Bible stories of Joseph reveal that he would have been justified for feeling bitter about the rejection by his family, his exile and years of imprisonment in Pharaoh's dungeon before becoming master of his fate. "But the critical question remains: When his past shows up unexpectedly at his palace door, will Joseph slam it shut, or open it wide in welcome?" writes Biblical scholar and psychotherapist Naomi Rosenblatt.

Caring for a parent throws open the door to our past and demands that we look at it squarely. The past cannot be changed; the future is ours to create. Despite any misgivings about our obligations, we are afraid of coming up short of both moral and social expectations. What we find is not so much that we are incapable, but that we are testing new limits, learning broader ways of being in the world. Growing up means opening up. We can only accomplish that in the faith that doing the right thing is a sacred mystery to be revealed in time.

Into the Abyss

In my nightmares, icy waves came curling toward shore, freezing into white maidens straining off the prow of a ghost ship. On gray sands I stood, a spectral witness watching my life undulate before me, unable to control the tide of crises. Afraid of not measuring up to what was required, unsure of what that even was at times, I was loath to ignore reality and doubly terrified to embrace it. But there was no turning back—and nothing to turn back to.

Here was hard truth, where hope demanded I put my faith in a will and purpose greater than my own. Among other problems, we were running out of money; only a miracle could stave the onslaught. The first came one spring day from the local Jewish welfare council. Their social worker, Melanie, had heard murmurings that my parents were in trouble. There was a small outreach account; would it be helpful? I unleashed so many emotions in that moment, reinvigorated by the concern of friends. There were two sticking points, however: the funds would cover only a couple of months' bills, and it would be nearly impossible to get Dad to accept help. Melanie offered to take their case by suggesting the money as a loan to cover prescriptions, which were averaging $700 a month. I thought perhaps the council might also sponsor a private fund-raiser. They agreed but admonished me to return to Wichita and work out a more stable care plan. So I did.

A thankful number of donations came in; timing could not have been better. Growing worse each week, my parents needed basic care at least twelve hours a day. Mother's medications had to be crushed several times a day and mixed into food, which had to be a certain consistency and temperature or she couldn't swallow. Since it was against regulations for a home chore worker to dispense drugs, either a family member or a licensed professional nurse had to do it—the latter at huge expense.

For a moment, care was stabilized. When I was ready to return to California, however, Father decided he needed surgery to implant a line that would dispense measured amounts of morphine. He had been enduring unfathomable pain for months, probably years, and had postponed the procedure, afraid to become addicted and unwilling to allow the implications. Surgery would take three to five days, so he asked if I would stay on.

Aunt Sam returned so that each parent could have attention. On a shimmering Wednesday the paramedics came for Father. Before they lifted him into the van, he asked them to pause: he hadn't been outside for nearly six months, and he wanted to inhale the sweet prairie breezes that made all things safe, all things known. After three days no doctor had visited, even though he had chosen this hospital on the other side of town because it was convenient to his physician. I called to complain vigorously, outraged by the lack of attention to a dying man and woman.

My father's stay escalated into two torturous weeks as a proper dosage to balance hallucinations with rational presence could not be stabilized. Mom was hysterical, phoning Dad twenty times a day and waking him so often that I had to cut her off from the one she loved most. Undaunted, she would somehow ready her next day's outfits, laying out a sharp cranberry wool suit with cream crepe blouse on one end of Dad's empty bed, a heather jacket and skirt with a pink ruffled polyester shirt at the other. It must have taken all night.

Father insisted I return home, not wanting to keep me from Bob and work. I wanted to stay; I even offered to move back indefinitely. "You are your mother's daughter," my father said out of nowhere, freeing me from the self-inflicted worry that I wasn't devoted enough. The morning of my departure Dad developed an infection. Now came a confusion of antibiotics and anti-seizure medication to prevent cardiac arrest from so much morphine. I insisted I must stay; I couldn't bear to leave him like that. As much as he had always protected me, however, he would not cling to me. I cried hysterically for days, even though the infection cleared.

The day before Dad left the hospital, while cradling Mom into the car, Sam slammed the door on her own hand. The pain was excruciating, exacerbated by ragged emotions. Crying all the way to the hospital and wanting sympathy but getting none, Sam deposited Mom in Dad's room and went for an X ray of her hand. The news was devastating: her caregiving days were over. But she wasn't the one who informed me; it was Melanie, who said that unless I could come right back and stay indefinitely, we would have to hire full-time help. Her health destroyed, my aunt had collapsed, complete with pneumonia. She could not bear to tell her brother the extent of her condition; she left soon after he returned home, tethered to bed and death and a wife who had no comprehension of the extent of their decline.

I wanted to save my parents, save us all, but the abyss swallowed me whole.

CHAPTER 5

Spousal Caregiving

Eighty-four thousand doors open to the truth of interbeing, and suffering is one of them. But there are also other doors, including joy and lovingkindness.—Thich Nhat Hanh

When a lifelong partner becomes ill, losses are great: companionship, dreams, security, and intimacy. "In sickness and in health" becomes not just an innocent wedding vow but a crucible of loyalty, a consecration of heart and soul. If we have no strong sense of self, we can disappear into the illness, caught up in the terror of what is to come, the loss of what went before.

Typically, the focus is on the one who is ill; the partner becomes a wallflower even though a mate's well-being resides in the partner's hands. "We're the people others usually look past, the people pushing the wheelchair," says one spouse whose husband has had multiple sclerosis for more than two decades. "When your spouse is ill, you lose your lover, your best friend, and the person you expected to grow old with. Your family cannot replace the loss that you have suffered."

The Specter of Loss

When we marry, we are blissfully ignorant of what it means to grow old together. As a couple we envision the ideal partnership—happy family, healthy children, active retirement. On the altar, despite our pledge, we don't consider what "till death" might require. And so we continue, until the unthinkable happens and the future blurs.

Although it is illogical, illness can feel like betrayal, a miscarriage of marital hopes and promises. The well spouse grows angry that so many years have been taken away and resents losing control over life. Whereas many systems are in place to help the one who is ill, healthy spouses often receive little support. Although it is expected that the spouse will take over, it is not an automatic skill. Established gender roles are overturned: the wife becomes the decisionmaker, the husband the homemaker. Especially for elderly couples, men find it more difficult to care for wives because traditionally it was the woman who did the child-raising and husband-tending. Because the well spouse is the primary caregiver almost half the time, often with no backup, he or she can soon reach the end of stamina. Then, if there is no other family to step in, a nursing home may seem like the worst violation of love and trust—the caregiver feels impossible guilt at not having been able to cope because of physical, emotional, or financial stresses.

"These are supposed to be the golden years," says Nancy Morrison, director of clinical services at a social services agency. "The kids are raised, you are toying with the idea of retirement, vacations—and now it's all back to ground zero." In a materialistic world we gather in and preserve those possessions and relations that define who we believe ourselves to be. Any threat to that collection is inconvenient at best, unbearable at worst. We have vested in a belief that nothing changes; yet as wisdom traditions—and life—teach, that is delusion.

For both caregiver and care receiver, losses are both real and imagined, from job and social position to friends, dignity, and physical abilities. Partnership itself changes as each layer of self is peeled back to reveal more than we may wish to have known. In caring for a spouse, we fulfill the true meaning of marital bonds as we are asked to extend ourselves under the most trying circumstances: we are asked to love unconditionally.

According to Maggie Strong, founder of the Well Spouse Foundation and caregiver for a husband with multiple sclerosis for more than twenty years, spousal caregiving differs from parent care in these critical ways:

~ The workload: Even though the ill person is doing all he or she can do, there's a constant sense of inequality. The spouse takes on many work roles—depending on the severity of the illness—and does so forever, so that leisure time vanishes and recuperation time vanishes. The work becomes second nature, so that it's a hard habit to break. It's hard to learn how to get what help you can from the ill spouse. Then, if you are giving hard-core nursing and hygiene care, that's an overwhelming combination.

~ Intimacy: There are very few chronic illnesses that yield a good sexual life—it's not like making love with the person you knew. A lot of coping is by abstinence, with the resulting pains; some decide to have something on the side and find it gets too complex emotionally—there is terrible guilt. This is not just an older person's issue. This can happen to people who are thirty years old. I know of a young woman whose husband fell off a roof and became a quadriplegic, and she is looking at forty more years of marriage. This is not what you meant when you said "I do."

~ Finances: If you need skilled aides or a nursing home, the rich can afford it; the poor have Medicaid. If you're a middle-class person, you're not going to remain a middle-class person to qualify for coverage.

~ Children: When one parent is limited and suffering and the other parent is filling in all the cracks, what's left for the kids? Not much, generally. Vacations are gone, attention is gone, variety is gone. Their belief that *their* problems matter is gone. Everything rotates around this illness. And kids are frightened: Will my parent die? Will I get it? There's just not enough to go around, and options are reduced.

~ Emotions: Caregiving takes so much energy—and you don't have much energy anymore. Your friends have fallen away, there is social isolation. A well spouse is neither married nor not married: you are an anomaly. You get angry; it's too frustrating. The American ideal is that things will get better. Things here get worse. This is a different place to live; if you don't live in it, you don't get it.

This is the hard-core reality of spousal caregiving, but we have a choice each minute whether to be a victim or to take responsibility for our feelings. To be a "poor baby" is not fate; it is a decision. And though it takes great discipline and intent to counter a tendency to feel sorry, we always have that power within us.

The Loss of Identity

"You bury it so deep," says Janet, who cared for Ray, her husband of fifty-two years, living his life for him, losing her own in him. In the beginning she didn't know what was happening; everybody forgets things. In the beginning, there was denial. Janet admits they went through a period of hate and resentment over all the craziness that dementia imposes.

She let Ray do for himself as long as he could; he would shave himself, sometimes for an hour. But then he began shaving the towel, so she took over. He never stopped moving; she could never slow down. Then he became incontinent, and she became responsible for his whole life. Bound to him alone in the house, she started to have a nervous breakdown. She didn't ask her daughters for help even though they knew what she was going through—it didn't seem right to have them change their father's diapers. "So I became him—I lost myself completely in those two years. I was my own worst enemy. But I took excellent care of him."

Eventually Ray fell and could not do well by himself any longer. Janet reluctantly placed him in a nursing home. She visited every day, walked him, fed him, flossed and brushed his teeth, changed his diaper, and put him down for a nap. For a year and a half she kept constant vigilance as Ray deteriorated. Then he contracted a urinary infection and they never got him back. He was eighty. At the end, his family was with him as well as the pastor and the granddaughters. Janet was holding his hand. He took his last breath and she was in awe. She didn't know it could be that way—the years of heartache and pain just ended. Death took all that away. But it was not over for Janet.

I could not get myself back for a long time after his death. It was like a breakdown—you don't know how to live, you don't know how to think straight. Your own life means nothing at all; you don't care if you live or die. I would look at people and think, "Oh, they're living, if only I could live that way." Sure they were walking around with their problems, too, and no one knew this was going on inside me, though the children saw some of it. I dedicated my life to him, and this was a part of my marriage. He needed help, he was a human being, but gradually he went away.

Loss of identity is experienced as a loss of self, says transpersonal philosopher Michael Washburn. "Usually our sense of being derives from our identity in the world, and therefore the loss of identity carries with it the feeling of loss of being, of death." It is a dying to the world as well, an alienation from established patterns and expectations. The self is consigned to a limbo; the former identity no longer has a home, and meaning is cast out with memorabilia. We become spectators of our lives, a seemingly hopeless situation. There is only yearning for a something not yet known—but it will appear when conditions are right and we find the road back home.

The Loss of Partnership

Especially in a disease that robs the mind, there is a great loss of companionship. But any debilitating illness foists survivor's guilt on the well spouse along with a sense of never-ending uncertainty. Harlan cares for his wife, Carol, who has been assaulted for almost a decade by chronic back pain. Only in their forties, they have searched extensively for diagnosis and relief—the myelogram, MRI, CAT scan, alternative therapies such as acupuncture and herbs—but with few answers. Carol is trying psychology-as-pathology therapy, which proposes that physical pain masks emotional problems, while Harlan is active in on-line caregiver support groups and the Well Spouse Foundation. Even though there have been flickers of progress, Carol is now considered disabled and qualifies for Social Security. But they keep searching.

"What's been so frustrating is that you can't figure out what it's about, and therefore you can't do anything about it," Harlan says. "By definition caregiving doesn't *affect* your life, it *becomes* your life. Outside activities disappear; your friends disappear. In eight years I have been to the movies three times. I could go more, but I'm at work all day and the last thing I want is to leave Carol alone more. And she can't sit long enough to go to a movie."

Harlan says the physical and logistical elements are easier than providing emotional support and feeling responsible for her self-esteem.

> When Carol's okay, she's a joy to be around—smart, funny, warm, compassionate. The problem is, she is not okay an awful lot of the time. What I've had to do more than anything is recognize my anger, because rationally you know this is nobody's fault. And you know that however bad you're feeling, she's feeling worse.
>
> My wife knows she's sick, and there's always the question, "Am I ever going to get better—or well?" It's a real purgatory place for both of us. We want off the roller coaster, but dumping her in a nursing home or divorce and remarriage are not among the possibilities. The great hope is we'll get back to a normal life. If we can't, then I hope she comes to terms with it in such a way that she can at least enjoy the life she has to the greatest level possible.

In caring for a spouse, we learn that only the present is given to us and that it is our choice how to react to it. We realize that no anchor exists in past or future but only in our integrity of the moment, beyond the agenda of selfhood. It is in the now that we live, and in the now that we can give.

Loss of Hearth and Home

It is both human nature and the nature of caregiving to feel that we alone must tend to all of our spouse's needs, always. Holding to that belief is a cause of inestimable stress; letting go of it is the window to coping. When we must give over care to a professional setting, there is great guilt and a period of empty adjustment to separation—from our spouse, from our heart's desire. But it can be done.

A constant sadness is always with Mary. It was a great loss when she had to place her husband, Bruce, in a nursing home. He cannot walk, he cannot speak, and he is incontinent after several seizures. The deterioration came gradually—with subtle changes in behavior, in confidence, in reasoning. Over ten years, Mary and their two supportive daughters watched Bruce close his little music shop, lose his ambition and his sense of self, as she took over fixing leaky faucets, refinancing the house, and doing the taxes. Mary thought it uncharacteristic of Bruce to sit at home while she continued teaching high school mathematics, and her heart hurt for him because he seemed frightened. But she suppressed her feelings, sharing them only with her children, who realized before their mother did that the changes appeared serious. One daughter asked Mary and Bruce to move from Tennessee closer to her in Washington.

Mary decided to retire, figuring Bruce wouldn't be so alone, and they could take walks together. Maybe, she thought, he might even snap out of it. So they relocated; less than two years later, Bruce began having seizures. Then he was diagnosed with probable Alzheimer's. Mary sought the advice of senior services, consulted with a lawyer, studied up on Medicaid eligibility in case Bruce had to go into a convalescent facility, which would cost $50,000 a year. She obtained durable powers of attorney and living wills for both of them—none too soon, as a few weeks later Bruce could no longer sign his name.

Today, Mary, now sixty-seven, visits the nursing home daily, still thinking of herself as a caregiver, never resentful for it. She greets Bruce with a hug and kiss, tells him how glad she is to see him in the tone of voice she has reserved for him for fifty-two years. She grooms him, takes him for a stroll in his wheelchair, washes his eyeglasses, watches TV or listens to classical music with him. She recently moved to a new house nearby and rents out their former home. Despite being at peace with her decision, she hates what has happened to Bruce, to their lives, losing the person who made her feel she was the apple of his eye.

I care for him deeply. My grief and depression are always present; I cry easily and I cry a lot. There are always reminders of what he once was—his guitar, his many stacks of choral music, his woodworking books, paper with his handwriting. One time when I opened the closet, there were his clothes. When I turned down the bed, there was his pillow, not to be slept on. In the bathroom was the place his towel always hung.

Despite her sorrow, Mary feels guilt only in wondering if Bruce might be uncomfortable, lonely, or sad. At seventy, he has been at the nursing facility for more than two years. But she has uncovered strengths she didn't know she had, and along with the joy she takes in her daughters and grandchildren, she hopes she is demonstrating loyalty to a loved one. "There are some very nice people in this world. Some of the staff members at the nursing home go beyond the call in their kindnesses and day-to-day caring. Their work is hard and often thankless; if there is a heaven, I think their crowns will be filled with stars."

We want to remain in our fairy tales forever, but catastrophic illness forces us to leave the land of make-believe. All is impermanent. It is our clingings and aversions, our resistance to change, that create suffering. By corollary, it is a patient heart that releases suffering, for it is not who we are when caregiving begins that defines our character and sets us free, but who we end up becoming.

Moving beyond Loss

For those who have overridden the sunny decrees of the everyday world to follow a call to relieve suffering, obstacles become openings, time and again. Sacred literature is filled with stories of this "exile," the best known being the turning out of Adam and Eve from Paradise and the forty-year wandering of the Israelites in Jewish lore, as well as the spiritual quest of Siddhartha in Buddhist mythology.

When Devara was thirty-five, she married the love of her life, Derek. He was eighteen years her senior and a superb recreational athlete. When he was fifty-nine he began to get cramps biking to work. They didn't subside, so the couple visited a neurologist, who delivered the verdict with a piercing blow: "Derek has Parkinson's and there's nothing I can do to save him."

Wanting a second opinion, they trekked a hundred miles to a famous neurologist, whom Devara found insensitive and arrogant. But when he conducted a simple exam to measure mental capabilities, Derek couldn't add twenty-five and ten, didn't know the day's date. She had a foreboding sense of doom; that night she wept in Derek's arms, for both him and their future. The diagnosis eventually was given as Parkinson's and dementia, but no one explained what that meant. So Devara, a pharmacist's daughter and former health researcher and planner, began to educate herself.

For the next four years she tried to be the perfect wife, friend, caregiver. As Derek's illness progressed, his cramps became more painful, and the dementia worsened. Still working and caretaking full time, Devara studied up on his medications and researched comfort care alternatives like faith healing, aromatherapy, acupuncture, physical therapy, and water therapy. She hung his sheets outside so the scent of fresh air could permeate his bedroom. She made sure he was well fed and comfortable and did everything she could think of, without support from family or medical professionals.

Eventually she took a leave of absence to care for Derek full time. Every day the diseases extracted a pinch more: a word was lost, an emotion vanished. He was becoming so frail, the time came when he couldn't even exercise in the pool. Then Devara's days grew terribly long. Every day she had to lift and carry him from their sunken living room to the bedroom, adding to her exhaustion and desolation. For eleven months she continued on this way, immersed in grief, sleeping three hours a night if at all.

Then she called a home health agency, which sent a marvelous nurse and wound specialist who took over some of the chores and taught needed skills: how to prepare low-cost nutritional shakes, how to change Derek's diaper without hurting him, how to change the dressing on a gaping bedsore. Most especially, she offered compassion and reaffirmed Devara's worth as a loving caregiver, something no one else had done.

But Devara already was becoming a danger to herself. When the time came for a wheelchair for Derek, she waged battle with the durable medical supply system, outraged at the lack of compassion and guidance. When she needed a ramp built indoors, it took fifteen calls to get an affordable contractor. When the wrong air mattress arrived, she became hysterical. When she had to fight insurance companies over home health coverage, she cracked.

"I became verbally and physically abusive to Derek. I was absolutely appalled because I was manifesting these behaviors that I would never in a sane moment manifest. I was watching myself do it and yet I was so out of control I couldn't stop. I couldn't believe I was being abusive to a vulnerable person—and worse, to the person I loved more than anyone in the world."

Rescuing strength from love, she pulled herself back from the brink. And when after a few days her tormented behaviors passed, she went out into their breezeway and had an epiphany: she vowed that not only would she regain control over her life, but she also would help other caregivers. And that is exactly what she has done, through lobbying and other advocacy work.

Ultimately, everything she went through, all the terrible fear and agony, ended up only in gratitude in the last moments. Derek died in her arms; Devara let him know he was loved, the greatest gift she could give.

I am so grateful that I was his caregiver, that he didn't die in a nursing home or in a hospital. And no matter how horrific that experience was—no one wants to go through war, no one wants to be a caregiver again—it is such a rewarding experience, it is such a spiritual experience, and it is such a rich experience. The dying process is not to be feared. We should embrace it.

We're a very immature culture; it's going to take a long time, but those of us who have gone through the fire can bring back this wisdom and information. Once we do that, we will have taken a major step into becoming mature, a truly wise society.

ACTION STEPS

~ Talk about illness and dying while you both are still healthy.

~ Create legal and financial documents that clearly state your wishes, including beneficiaries, and update them every few years and/or when there is a change in family composition.

- ~ Make inventories of all your important possessions, such as jewelry, electronics, photographs, and collections.
- ~ Learn to identify uncomfortable emotions and to talk about them so that hurts and misunderstandings don't fester.
- ~ Tell your children where your important papers are kept. Discuss estate matters and end-of-life issues before a crisis hits.
- ~ Delegate responsibilities so that you can retain the more important aspects of your partnership without fatigue or resentment.
- ~ Use the Internet to develop support networks and to educate yourself, or as a supplement to local support groups.
- ~ Remember that your children still need the attention of parents. Involve them in the illness and care plan so they know you all are still a family despite disruptions.

Out of the heartache of caring for a partner come lessons and survivorship skills that inform a lifetime and set examples for the next generation. Reality can be brutal, but it is also conditioned by attitude. Even if we have been stripped of one set of dreams, we can choose how we will respond at each moment, and can turn tragedy into an adventure made together, for all time.

Perhaps we have not so much left home when we are called upon to change our familiar ways as we have been asked to open ourselves to life. To love, honor, and cherish are easy words on days of celebration; sorrowful promises in the face of chronic illness. In marriage we vow to become one. In so doing, our identities, our dreams, and our greatest joys wrap around its promise. When illness wedges into this most private relationship, we are challenged to find ways to cope with loss—but also to reweave a new matrix. For the common threads are love, which needs no form, and compassion, which needs no permission.

Do Not Resuscitate

"Your poor father—he's really broken down."

The words stung; the social worker, Melanie, spared no feelings. "He's a lot different than when he went into the hospital; he knows the drugs are masking his mental status." Melanie called my parents' situation a nightmare, but vowed to do as much as she could, clearly expecting me to look into a nursing home—and quickly, despite my exhaustion, ignorance, and distance. We scrambled to arrange care. Home health aides from a reputable agency were dispatched to perform some light housekeeping and personal assistance.

Clara, the aide, agreed to increase her work load from fifteen to forty hours a week, at $6 an hour. My parents also engaged Emily, a former housekeeper who had remained like family. She would work the eight- to ten-hour overnight shifts at an additional $500 a week. At these rates it looked like we had enough pooled funds to keep them at home only four to six more weeks.

Father acquiesced to reality: he finally agreed to elect Medicare's hospice benefit for both of them. Immediately their outlay for medicine was reduced to $5 co-payments; they had aides and volunteers a few hours a week, an additional social worker, and regular at-home skilled care. Their primary nurse, Nancy, was my lifeline. Her respect, calm, and graciousness were endearing.

The truth was numbing, however: Mother was sleepless and anxious, choking more because of increased salivation. She also refused bathing and having her blood pressure tested, so Medicare stopped coverage for home care. Dad could no longer get out of bed, and despite intensified dosages of morphine he was wracked with pain. Boosters caused hallucinations and hot flashes. The drugs made him so nauseated that he was losing weight from lack of appetite.

Troubles tumbled in one after another. Emily soon quit, unable to abide the torrent of problems in people she loved. Clara also considered leaving unless she got more money, but then she became gravely ill and wound up hospitalized. Dad wanted his sister to return, but she was not well enough. Melanie insisted on creative and serious planning because Father, in an effort to remain in control, was interfering with schedules by canceling shifts at the last minute, resisting efforts to let the professionals manage their lives.

Against a roar of inner voices, I found no refuge except in my husband's generous spirit. By day I was given no time off work; by night I clambered to the window gasping for air. I felt misunderstood, isolated. I needed so much more reassurance than friends or colleagues could give, despite their best efforts. I dreaded asking for another leave of absence but I had to go home again. Winging back across the Continental Divide, I sank into a schizophrenic existence.

One night Father asked me to help pay the bills. For the first time I understood the magnitude of their plight—the second mortgage to finance the foundering insurance business with my uncle, the borrowing against credit cards to finance home health—always one step ahead of disaster. I saw only one option, as we all were careening into bankruptcy: to take the private fund-raising for home care into the community.

One night, from my father's expansive basement library, I called the mayor, a friend of my parents after Father managed his successful campaign. I knew I was in a privileged situation—not everyone knows a mayor—but I was desperate for help. I went behind my parents' backs, reasoning that welfare would be a worse indignity than public knowledge of their distress. The mayor's hesitation proclaimed both astonishment and shame, for not knowing the dire situation and for having believed Father, who always assured everyone they were fine. The mayor agreed it was time for the city to give back to my parents and vowed to be the white knight to make it happen.

When everything was as stable as I could make it, for the fourth time in eight months I said good-bye to my parents, ever more certain these would be our final hugs and kisses. I left them in the morning, their "Do Not Resuscitate" window sticker the last thing I saw as I closed the door. Half a nation away from my husband Bob's comforting arms, I entered pandemonium. But the golden wheat fields, wide expanses, and sweet prairie gentleness consoled my soul, assuring me that this kind land would welcome my parents back.

Energized once again by traveling past crimson sunsets, I knew that when all had been said and done, the earth and the stars would be waiting for me, healing my wounds and giving them meaning. *Ad astra per aspera* (to the stars through difficulty), Kansas's state motto, was my childhood mantra. Now it would guide me home.

PART II

Emotional Wilderness

CHAPTER 6

The Nature of Loss

When her firstborn child died in infancy, she was griefstricken. Carrying his body everywhere, she roamed the streets, begging to find a holy man to perform a miracle and restore his life. Eventually she visited the Buddha, who told her to go into the city and bring back a mustard seed from any house in which there had never been a death. For weeks she wandered, at last understanding the lesson: the one law of the universe is impermanence; accepting death can free us from suffering.—A Buddhist tale

Whether it happens imperceptibly over time or in the flash of crisis, family caregiving refocuses lives, severing those involved from familiar patterns and thrusting them into a land unknown, where human fears prey on the unsuspecting. Yet it is also fertile ground, where detachment from the past allows a new destiny to take root. Seen from the outside, one loss rolls off another. But from within, caregiving can be the life-altering event by which a person shifts direction from linear concerns of the rational mind to the abstract promptings of the inner world, a turning from the ephemera of society to the calling of the soul.

In universal archetype, a crisis compels the unsuspecting hero to leave his everyday realm for one less common—the psyche—and to confront the phantoms of his past: the orphan dreams and desires that were cast away so many years before but that still rumble with life. A Greek legend powerfully elucidates this journey of separation and loss and the way back to wholeness: if you were traveling to Athens, the road to success, you had to pass by Procrustes and be placed on his bed. Any part of you that was too long would get lobbed off; if you were too short, you got stretched.

We are socialized into a mold of what is normal, right, and best—cut off from our true voice when an aspect of ourselves is rejected or doesn't measure up to one-size-fits-all expectations. All parts of us remain somewhere; the hidden pieces are still linked to us. The task is to recover them and restore balance so that the ordained fears can no longer overtake us. In caregiving, when so much wisdom is required, it is time to listen to those feelings of guilt and helplessness, inadequacy and depression. It is time to bring loss into the light of wisdom so that we will see our separation as illusion and our lives as fluidity. It is time to understand the nature of loss and our power over it.

"We must allow ourselves to feel the loss and letting go. . . . There is no way to avoid the transitions of life. The chief means of entering them gracefully is to practice them mindfully over and over again," writes Buddhist meditation teacher Jack Kornfield in *A Path with Heart*. Family caregiving is such an odyssey, into an emotional wilderness where roles and identities, beliefs and desires, are stripped away by the demands of a strange new calling. We meander over these changes in our personal landscape, looking for road signs to tell us where we are now and where we are heading.

This is the moment of truth: we are all beings who are going to die. We want to flee this demon awareness but cannot, for we have been called to serve. We have no choice but to venture into this ominous truth. We enter what theological mystic St. John of the Cross illumines as a period of withdrawal that cleanses the habits that have hidden the indwelling spirit. It is a phase inescapable to any soul wishing to be free, a dying to the world and death of the self—known in Zen as the great doubt, in Islam as the state of self-accusing. St. John explained:

Although this happy night brings darkness to the spirit, it does so only to give it light in everything; and that, although it humbles it and makes it miserable, it does so only to exalt it and raise it up; and although it impoverishes it and empties it of all natural affection and attachment, it does so only that it may enable it to stretch forward, divinely, and thus to have fruition and experience of all things, both above and below.

This stage is part of the inner journey: we sway between illumination and impotence in preparation for surrender of self. What appears to be barren is merely dormant, waiting to be wakened. This boundary between old and new states of being melts away cherished dross and leaves us to encounter mortality, often for the first time. Yet these growing pains are a fruitful darkness, says anthropologist Joan Halifax, a threshold when the limits of self are recognized and tested—and broken.

Change is often unwelcome, but it announces its true nature under psychic duress. Says Buddhist meditation master Sogyal Rinpoche:

It is only when we believe things to be permanent that we shut off the possibility of learning from change. . . . Grasping is the source of all our problems. Since impermanence to us spells anguish, we grasp on to things desperately, even though all things change. We are terrified of letting go, terrified, in fact, of living at all, since *learning to live is learning to let go.*

The Cycles of Grief and Mourning

"Grief goes in cycles, like the seasons, like the moon," writes Hope Edelman in *Motherless Daughters*. With every change in a loved one's functional ability, a caregiver mourns. Grief is not limited to death: it is also about losing capacity—to write checks, to drive, to cook, to remember birthdays—as well as about expectations of certain results.

Just as grief involves stages that feel like implosions, it also begets new wisdom skills. "Adult life brings its own spiritual tasks and openings," says Jack Kornfield. "Each stage of life holds the seeds for our spiritual growth. Our spiritual life matures when we consciously accept the life tasks appropriate for us . . . the spiritual tasks that require our heart to grow in commitment, fearlessness, patience, and attention." Endings remind us of other beginnings, like the surprises in our garden, each in due season. Although they feel like loss to the personality, these sheddings are victory to the soul.

In a death-denying culture, we are swimming against the tide, convinced of our own pathology. We're a fix-it society—we like smiling faces and happy, active people, says Lee L. Pollak, a licensed clinical social worker who coordinates bereavement programs for Jewish Family and Children's Services.

> There's not a lot of room for the devastating sadness that comes with grief. Society has a way of ignoring cycles of crying and immobilization, making people feel they should get on with it after a set time. That's a disservice, because there's a huge range of normal feelings that people experience when dealing with loss and different kinds of grief. There's situational grief that follows a death, and the grief that comes as people go through the transformations of aging and different stages of their lives. The more complicated the relations, the more complicated the grief reaction will be. And with greater longevity—seniors today never expected to live this long or be this healthy—people can expect to go through many more stages than in the past.
>
> Even if it's a good loss, change always means leaving something and hopefully starting something new. Not all stress is distress, but we don't do a good job of saying good-bye to one stage before moving on. Dealing with loss is not forgetting but learning how to integrate it and move forward.

Grief is initiation into an undiscovered country, a casting off of attachments to the outer world to find mooring within. It exacts a shift in consciousness, permission to step onto a less traveled path. It is a psychological ungluing, the bewilderment of not knowing how or if the situation will ever be resolved; yet there is a determination to keep going. We have engaged on a path and it will change us, but now we are more willing.

The Path of Initiation

The quintessential "call to adventure" of mythology can occur at any stage of adulthood, but it descends poignantly when we confront death, most commonly around middle age. Life is suddenly larger, and former ways seem constricting. "What used to feel secure and comforting now feels life-denying, and suddenly we know it is time to leave home," writes psychologist Sherry Ruth Anderson in *The Feminine Face of God*. What it feels like now is "not knowing." So we must find the place that knows.

This stage requires a crossing from lower to higher self, from personality- to soul-directed behavior. To the ego it is a fearful place— for at the gate of awareness the dweller on the threshold must lose her- or himself by merging with what theosophy calls the angel of the presence. This union of divine and human is called illumination or initiation, a transformation that leads out of self-absorption and into spiritual rebirth toward a life of service. It is liberation from control by the lower nature, but with it comes responsibility of a more selfless order.

One must give up the glamors of ignorance and self-pity to meet the unlived spiritual life. The Greek name for this path is *katabasis*, or descent into the psyche; it signifies deep introspection, a mourning of lost youth or dreams. This course appears to be a hazardous route where unseen forces conspire to strip away self-importance and other reflections of the ego, humbling us and opening our vision beyond personal pursuits. As we venture within we are shocked by how painfully long we've turned away from wholeness and from the joy of unshakable certainty. We have been preoccupied with outer nibblings, believing in limitation and evading the shadowy emotions that lead to the "certainty of the View" of Tibetan Buddhism.

The impact of being *here* now, of being forced by circumstance to pay attention to these uninhabited parts of ourselves that demand restitution, is bewildering as we encounter rage, betrayal, despair, and bitterness. Since childhood these emotions have remained there, waiting for our return. In the interim, they have gained power. Caregiving forces us to reexamine our motives and, for self-preservation, to withdraw to the realm where wisdom and compassion are whole and accessible. Author Sophy Burnham calls it "the second journey," not the one of rational reality but that which pierces the gossamer veil between secular and spiritual. It is a metamorphosis, a process of continual transformation as the journeyer probes further into the mysteries of life and death, assimilating them and then transcending viewpoint after viewpoint.

Eileen, a hospice director, has worked near death for more than twenty years. For five years she cared for her mother, who battled Alzheimer's and seizures, in the midst of which her father, who is now ninety-three and lives with her family, suffered a stroke. She was caught in a whirlwind of finding new housing and medical care for both parents, missing out on her sons' birthday parties, feeling guilty that her mother's needs were consuming her, but knowing that was how it had to be. After her mother died, Eileen, fifty-one, experienced grief as a spiritual mandate.

Recently she was pummeled by news that her husband, Maurice, sixty-one, has gastric cancer; they thought it was a persistent stomach flu. Initially his prognosis was two years, but the wheel turned again: only a few weeks at best. Even with her working knowledge of seriously ill people, Eileen says, still the most difficult part is the unknown, the uncertainty even on just a practical level: Will Maurice return to work? What about their income with one child going off to college? Everything has become twisted, one knot after another.

The couple and their two boys, ages nine and seventeen, have refocused their energies: give Maurice every opportunity to beat the disease. Even though the doctors don't know who Eileen's family is or how they live, even though they have made assumptions, they understand this is a team. Eileen is taking care of the nuts-and-bolts queries, gathering reading material, and mobilizing a support network, while Maurice is concentrating on getting through the energy-stripping chemotherapy.

Eileen's overriding sorrow is that her husband of twenty-nine years has changed so much physically, losing his strength and agility. A former dancer with the San Francisco Ballet, he has always been vibrant, active, and passionate about people. He has been a teacher of English as a second language for twenty-five years and a poet and sketch artist. To their sons he is still "Poppy"; there is no regret, only honesty and acceptance. Yet it is still a shock. Maurice has lost fifty pounds; it is difficult to eat despite his love of good food.

Even with a large, rich network of professionals and friends for which they are grateful, at times Eileen is confused and isolated. No matter how much support is there, she still feels cut off from something—"from the future, a livelihood, the ability to grow old with someone."

> Our life has changed, but Maurice and I essentially have not changed. We see to it that we keep the boys' schedule going, but it's new territory; it's the long-term stuff that fills me with fear. But after twenty years in hospice, after experiencing so much death, it informs you in a special way like nothing else can. It informs your every action, your ability to enjoy life; it informs the benchmarks of your life. Grief is like a big ocean wave: it just takes you out. Each time you go out, you don't know exactly when you're going to get back. And there are times I have felt absolutely shipwrecked. Yet every day with Maurice is a gift. We welcome the truth. It comes down to being an active observer, the witness: "What can I do for you?" Just be here, simply be here.
>
> If you allow grief in, there's nothing like it. Anyone can do it, be available to it. Just consider it—just consider it. And then you get swept away by it, and it deepens you like nothing else.

It is natural to feel overwhelmed and out of control—to not even know what or how to feel at all. There is nothing wrong with this state. The question is, how do you allow grief to happen so you can have healing at the same time? How do you make room for the emptiness? In more than two decades as a grief therapist, author Alexandra Kennedy has born witness to the prodigal process of going out and coming back, the transition back into daily reality after profound loss. Of the spiritual possibilities she says:

> We live in a culture where we don't deal with emptiness well. It is difficult to allow for that sense of space; we tend to want to get

away from it. There's a lot of pressure from jobs and friends and spouses to spring back to who you were, but you've changed. Now you're carrying grief, and it's a difficult time ahead. We need to take time daily to allow the not-knowing and the sense that our hands are empty and there's nothing more to do.

The quiet time alone to be with grief, what I call "sanctuary," allows the caregiver to explore the changes in values, questioning what matters and working out the unfinished business of relationship with the loved one. Are you willing to sit long enough for this new identity to emerge, or grab at the first thing because it's so uncomfortable you want to fill it up? If so, you sell yourself short. Grief is a transformational process that makes possible huge shifts in who you are. You emerge so much bigger than who you thought you were, but you won't get there if you don't go through the feeling that you've lost yourself. It is a very delicate time; the identity builds again very, very slowly on all the emotions surfacing through grief.

It's okay to feel empty and alone and to not know who you are and where you're going. You begin to build the seeds of a new life and you emerge with some sort of idea or creativity that is seeking to be expressed. It's a much fuller place because it receives so much more of life. It's almost as if our loved ones, in their deaths, give us the gift of life—again. And it's our choice if we take it, the second time.

Death Is a Mystery

Dying is a mystery, says Ram Dass, a pioneer in the field of mindful living since the early 1960s.

So you have to ask yourself, how do I deal with a mystery? Do I contract and push against it because it scares me too much? Or would I rather spend the last part of my life loving the mystery, embracing the mystery, realizing that the mystery of death increases the intensity and quality of my life?

As a caregiver, you're very concerned about the quality of life of your patient—but what about the quality of your own life? There are things you can do inside your own mind to change the quality of your life without changing the form of it. You still go to work, go through the same paces, but you find a place inside yourself that makes the entire experience different. The secret is coming into the moment—not living in the future or the past, but just being in the moment.

When a patient or loved one dies we are faced with the process of grieving. Often we get caught between the two ends of the cultural grieving syndrome. One is to keep a stiff upper lip, to get over it quickly and get on with life; the other is to become a professional griever, focusing on what we have lost. Between those two poles, you can feel a certain rhythm of grieving, and it happens at a different pace for different people. Our life structures have been built around the person who died, and that creates a continuous reminder of the absence of the other. You're used to knowing yourself through mirroring against your partner, for example, and suddenly you don't have that anymore. It takes time to find our way through that process.

When we've finished our grieving, we often come to a place where we are infused with the feeling of love that we had with the person who died, rather than with their loss. If we have touched another human being in love—in real love—it transcends death. Love has nothing to do with death, but as long as we're busy with our psychological losses, we can't quiet down enough to allow ourselves to see that nobody went anywhere. I've watched it happen again and again: when people finish with their grieving, they recognize that they haven't lost the essence of the relationship. They lost something, but it wasn't the essence of what they had with the other person. The communion is always there.

Though the world seems wind-washed and worn, it is possible to bear the unbearable. In the present moment there is no attachment; there is no fear. The mind lives in both past and future; the heart and its joy exist only in the infinite now.

In the mystical Shambhala, a hidden kingdom of enlightened

warriors found fulfillment and prosperity following principles of lovingkindness and fearlessness. To enter this peaceable place, caregivers must realize that the grief inherent in caring for a vulnerable love reveals a broader, cleaner vision of what matters, even if the objective world has not changed one bit. Here is the possibility of equanimity, a means for handling life's vicissitudes and remaining whole, long after caregiving is over.

It is our choice, in each of these nows, whether to participate fully in joy and sorrow or to turn away. It is within our power not to possess but to experience, not to hold but to embrace. This is how we transform loss: to be willing to stay open in the midst of suffering, to be strengthened rather than extinguished by it. When we choose an understanding heart, there is no more clinging to that which dies, but merging with that which loves. Out of this union we live again.

CHAPTER 7

The Stresses of Caregiving

What is truly merciful changes from day to day, even from
hour to hour. Often, we have to go to the extremes of
doing too much or too little for someone before we can
find the "right extent" of helping.—Wendy Lustbader,
Counting on Kindness

Family caregiving is one of the most stressful endeavors we may
ever engage in. Time was when such tasks could be a caregiver's
sole focus, but with women entering the workforce in large
numbers over the past twenty years, with new roles at home for both
men and women, with long-distance families, and with relatives who
are living longer, it's harder to balance it all today.

Snared by competing demands on time and energy, by perceptions of burden, and by fears for the future, at some time virtually
all caregivers suffer distress such as loneliness, exhaustion, anxiety,
and sadness. If unaddressed, these emotions can lead to severe disturbances including heart attacks, compromised immune systems, even
death.

Yet these feelings can be allies that reflect back the resistances that
need more attention and more understanding. It is not the number of

stresses but the coping and problem-solving skills that can make the difference between staying in balance and suffering from dysfunctional anxieties, between growing from the challenges or remaining mired in negativity.

Stress and Anxiety

"Just going through a terminal illness with a loved one can bring up its own difficulties," says Dr. Therese A. Rando, clinical director and founder of The Institute for the Study and Treatment of Loss in Warwick, Rhode Island. "Watching a loved one fade away or seeing horrific sights, being put in a situation of making choices, taking care of a person who is dying as well as other living people, trying to let go and hold on at the same time . . . this is traumatic stress."

So much stress comes from holding on to how we wish things were. Accustomed to snips of commitment rather than to attentive engagement, we become anxious when situations are more complicated than we thought. Making problems personal, we overreact or exaggerate, which clouds our judgment and blocks solutions that may be at hand. Because caregiving extracts us from our workaday pace and demands that we slow down, we may resent the forced change in lifestyle. The ensuing conflict produces emotions we seem unable to prevent or control, from denial of problems to arrogance that we alone are enough to tackle everything.

"The classic situation is that people get snared in the crisis and wait too long before they seek help. They get into caregiving assuming it's the short term. They put the crisis fire out and assume life will go back to the way it was," says Steve Rickards, former director of a senior and family support services program. "But it will never go back. Most caregiving is for the long term."

Professional case workers and medical professionals treat countless family caregivers who have worked themselves into the ground. They have not set limits or priorities nor delegated tasks; they have become so engulfed in caring that the snowball has become an avalanche. Geraldine Hall, a gerontology clinical nurse specialist with the Mayo Clinic in Scottsdale, Arizona, explains:

The major stressors stem from a continuing sense of loss of a loved one: of a relationship, of a lifestyle, of predictability, of autonomy, of roles of both caregiver and recipient. There is also loss of social status, financial security, and health. Add to this a sense of isolation, inadequacy, and rising family conflict. Add the fear of death and disability and a loss of companionship—it's a very, very complex issue.

There is also the fear of social sanction, belief that the marital vows preclude seeking help, fear of having strangers in the home, fear of abuse, concerns about loss of privacy, fear of crime with hired help, sanctions by family who do not understand the situation, poorly trained or inaccessible health and respite providers. When the burden becomes too great, our health breaks down; or when the sheer volume of care is too great, placement in nursing homes occurs. I have seen families, friends, clergy, the media, and public figures treat caregivers with great disdain, accusing them of abandonment, of using placement for convenience.

We expect people to rise to the most heroic tasks—to endure providing personal care for people who no longer recognize us, who soil themselves, fight care, become irrational and unreasonable—and often they do. The human spirit is capable of immeasurable love, hate, hope, despair—and stubborn tenacity.

Fear for the future and distress over being able to hold out are the undercurrent of caregiving. It takes great effort to keep loved ones autonomous, to provide the most dignified and loving care possible. The sense of deprivation, the not knowing, is a relentless source of anxiety.

"There are two faces to caregiver stress: it may be easier to bear the physical weight than the emotional burden of a seventy-five-year-old spouse unable to control her bladder," says Daniel Paris, a clinical social worker specializing in Alzheimer's. At this stage of the caregiving journey, both the physical and the emotional stresses are equal partners.

We need not be at the mercy of our shortcomings: we can train ourselves to be positive. A study by Ohio State University psychologists found that the power of negative thinking may have greater influence on well-being than the power of positive thinking. Further, those who spent a lot of time taking care of an ailing relative were more likely to be pessimists than those who did not, suggesting that a person's outlook may be more beneficial or harmful than the event itself.

The Problem of Isolation

One caregiver is worn out by unremitting loneliness. "This week I have really been feeling my isolation as a caregiver. My life is so full either of taking care of Mom or taking care of me so that I can continue to take care of her and still do my work. I am in a transition time with friends. I have recently lost some, and the new ones haven't appeared to replace them yet. So here I am, desperately needing some people in my life who can nurture me, and they're not around. And I don't have the time or energy to go out into social situations to meet new people. I need love and support."

This woman expresses a universal distress reaction: a breakdown of feeling connected. In a large survey of caregivers, the sense of isolation and the lack of understanding from others were reported as the most endemic problems caregivers face. Friends and relatives may be uncomfortable with a discussion of illness or death and avoid it; others may not know how to broach the subject or assume the caregiver doesn't want to talk about it. Oftentimes people *do* offer help, but caregivers, not wanting to bother them, don't respond. Those who are not involved cannot understand how hard caregiving is and may not offer consolation. Others may not know how to help or are waiting to be asked. If they are not included, they drift away.

Caregiving is not intentionally isolating, and yet it seems difficult to avoid some withdrawal if we want to do our best. Because caregivers solemnly believe they must do everything themselves, they assume no one can do it as well. This presumption poses a grave risk to all concerned. Scientific studies show that loneliness and isolation increase the risk of disease and premature death by 200 to 500 percent. When a caregiver becomes incapacitated, more than one life is compromised.

For months and with a clear measure of guilt, Barbara, sixty-eight, was in torment over placing her husband in a nursing home. Although she was wrung out, she worried that she was doing all she could, putting loyalty to their fifty years above her own health. She damaged her back by continually lifting Cy off the floor after he had slipped from the couch, cleaning carpets after his bouts with incontinence ten times a day. Still, she didn't feel she could ask for help, even from her daughters. Only after Cy suffered several small strokes and doctors said he would never get better did Barbara give up her watch and place him in a nursing home.

> I thought that no one could take care of him as well as I could, but staff members do. They keep him comfortable and clean. He even has a cup of coffee every morning with the administrator, and they let him attend staff meetings. I don't know what he does there, but he was a builder, and maybe he contributes something. This is his neighborhood now, and I feel like he's a person there. Life is quite different—I have never lived alone before—but I am surviving well.

Truth is, others will give good, but different, care. Caregiving is already a lonely business in a society frightened by wrinkles and illness, but that is exacerbated when we push ourselves to fulfill unrealistic hopes. Everyone has a right to his or her own life, and discovering that life is the inner journey of caregiving. Having confused loneliness with solitude, emptiness with loss, we need this time for introspection. Although we are in a stressful place, we are instructed by legend and myth that this is not true exile but wider perspective. Buddhist scholar Joanna Macy teaches that pain and despair and the lack of connectedness come from failure to recognize the world and its creatures as extensions of ourselves. Studying our aloneness, we discover the meaning of relationship; in the solitude of caring, we gain compassion for ourselves and fill a world of silences.

Guilt

Mimi Goodrich, a licensed clinical social worker and support group leader, identifies five hurdles that hinder most family caretaking: guilt, anger, denial, role changes, and confronting mortality. Of these, guilt is the most pervasive. "It's right up there for the adult child, feeling it's their obligation to make these years the happiest. But none of us has that power. When caregivers have expectations that are unrealistic, that's when the guilt comes in, saying, 'I should be able to do this.' "

There are many subtle ways we allow guilt in. "I have had many hurdles to jump in the last fifteen years," recalls Millie, sixty-five, who cared for her mother nonstop for three years in her own home.

It was hard to see my mother helpless and depending on me. I was homebound with her; day and night I had no life of my own. I had a husband but had to neglect things that we could do together. Then when she did die, I felt a relief and oh-so-guilty for that feeling. The guilt almost ate me up for a long time. Sometimes we feel guilty because we didn't spend as much time with our loved ones as we could. Or we feel guilty because we put them in a convalescent hospital or for a million different reasons.

But knowing that I kept her home and gave her the care she needed lifted me and made me truly realize the importance of having loved ones in my life. I knew that she needed to die, and I had the right to my life. I gave her all of me and more. The most important thing is that we stop and look at the overall picture and realize that we rejoice in the part that we know is for the betterment of everyone. The door that closes sometimes brings on a lot of pain, but pain is a part of life.

Guilt can tarnish even the best of situations. With her older sister Lynn, Barbara was caregiver to her mother, Marion, for a brief but intense period. Although Lynn is at peace, Barbara isn't as certain. "In reality we probably did enough, but this is the way I deal with things . . . I'm more emotional. I wonder if I really did enough." Barbara thinks back, says she could have let Marion stay at her house more often. Yet at the time her son was two and a half, and her husband is a therapist who works at home in the converted guest room. Barbara says maybe she could have spent some nights at her mother's, but after fourteen years of infertility and eight miscarriages, she finally had a son and wanted to be home with him.

It was hard when Marion went into the nursing home. Even though her mother died five days later, Barbara says, she didn't visit often enough. "It's hard to separate reality—'enough' is different for different people. If I had done things that made the rest of my life not make sense, maybe then I was doing enough for her, but not enough for me."

It is perhaps human nature that no matter how much a caregiver does for a loved one, it is hard to resolve the dilemma of not being able to do it all, especially to reverse fate. Unable to control everything and satisfy social convention, we feel we have not done enough. Guilt is not inherent—it is something we take on, and therefore something we can refuse. Our best *is* good enough. There is no way to give more than that.

Anger and Resentment

"Caregivers don't live in laboratories and clinics, they live in the real world." This statement comes from Stanford University researcher Abby King, whose first-of-a-kind study revealed that caring for relatives with mind-robbing diseases is more stressful for daughters than for wives, resulting in higher blood pressure and racing hearts. In psychological studies, daughters showed more resentment, anger, and a sense of being trapped. Why? Most children don't expect to be in this role; wives have the greater sense of duty as part of their marital vows.

No longer a child yet bonded to childhood wishes of how things should be, a daughter-caregiver can feel disoriented by what is being asked of her. As well, suggests Dr. Leonard Pearlin, professor of sociology at the University of Maryland, daughters are more likely to be burdened with family and job than a wife caring for an elderly husband. Daughters must also deal with conflicts among siblings who disagree about their roles.

For forty-one-year-old Becky, agonies go unabated as she tries to balance care for her mother with a father she wants to avoid. She volleys between anger over his unwillingness to extend himself to ease his wife's travails and a determination to extract every bit of tenderness from time with her mother, Amelia, who is seventy-eight.

Heartstricken over her mother's vascular dementia and furious toward her father, she lives in limbo. "Just about everything about this disease upsets me. I hate my life. Either I don't have enough time for Mom, or I don't have enough time for me. I have no friends anymore because everyone thinks I am crazy for spending all my free evenings with her and all day Saturdays as well," she says.

A medical librarian, Becky admires Amelia and shares her love of the arts. She spends more than twenty hours a week with her watching videos of opera, classical music, and dance and reading great literary works. Becky takes Prozac for depression and anger, anxious that she is not the ideal daughter. She admits feeling sorry for herself and her mother but not for her father, who demands attention but ignores his wife of fifty years. Becky is so tired, so filled with rage that seems to be as much a part of her as her skin. There is no relief in sight; Becky has been unable to get past her feelings.

> I am stumbling in the dark. I already feel bad not being able to offer my mom any cure, and that makes me feel helpless and worthless. I miss the mom who used to do crossword puzzles, who used to read the classics to me—Robert Louis Stevenson, Poe, Kipling. I tripped over her feet last night and fell backward but was not hurt. I shouted "Damnit," and so she cried and wanted to kiss my head. How can anyone prepare for the death of a parent, especially a loved parent?

It is not that emotions are not real; it is that we allow them the power to paralyze. We can move forward, but it takes commitment and choice. If all we can feel is sorry for ourselves, we will remain stuck in habits that drain and warp us. If we can take ourselves out of the equation even just one step, then our heartache will begin to soften. Coping skills can be developed and our responses to stress identified and defused.

Feeling Helpless or Frustrated

According to a survey by the National Family Caregivers Association, helplessness and frustration are two of the most common emotions on this path. Sometimes they are brought on by dealings with the health care system; other times they well up from life itself. Left to multiply unchecked, they can take over that life, even after the loved one has died. Faith, who recently lost her husband, Fred, is still in the throes of wondering when she will feel whole again. A longtime career woman whose accomplishments include counseling juveniles in the California Youth Authority State School for Girls and working with young people, she is shocked by the changes in herself.

> In just four months I've gone from a woman who could take almost anything in stride—caring twenty-four hours a day for her love, maintaining a house, seeing to repairs, nursing and nurturing him, shopping on the fly so as to not be gone too long, cooking, planning outings to a restaurant or concert in the park, sleeping with one ear open so if he moved I could be there to pick him up or call the paramedics—to this, where I feel almost helpless in my need for him.

Faith retired at age sixty-two so that she and Fred could enjoy their freedom; he had retired many years earlier. It was a second marriage for both. They were in their middle years but were so drawn to each other that their romance lasted twenty-seven years. Like a fool, she says, she thought it would go on forever. He never let a day go by without telling her how much he admired her ability on anything, how great she was—how lucky he was. There was always something nice to be said, but now there is only silence, deafening silence. Faith can't stand whining, but that doesn't erase the deep missing she is sure will go on forever.

Faith says that the five years of care for Fred, who had bleeding ulcers, dementia, and serious prostate problems, were like a seesaw of hope and despair and guilt that her best was not good enough to keep him alive. At first the deterioration came on gradually, but in his last few weeks, horrendously. With each change he would hold his head in his hands and say he couldn't bear it anymore. He died in Faith's arms with tears in his eyes, trying so hard to tell her something she couldn't understand.

Faith's bereavement has been colored by her disdain for the professionals entrusted with his care. She never heard from the doctors Fred was seeing at the time of his death, nor when she needed help with nutrition for a man who weighed less than one hundred pounds on his final day. She feels she was not treated as an equal partner but instead as a nuisance, wanting things that no one felt it necessary to give Fred. She hoped she was doing all she could, but vital information was not offered despite many pleadings to organizations for help.

> I got nothing practical to take home with me that said, "This will help you do better in giving care to this beloved person." I was drowning in confusion about my ability to do what had to be done. Some have told me that even after many years they revert to suffering and grief at unexpected times. But they say where there's life, there's hope, so I suppose we have only that to go on. It's a long, strange journey. Perhaps if I can work through this, eventually I will find some purpose that will give my life a sense of fulfillment.

Stress can be overwhelming, but it is the continual working through of these sorrows that leads out of them. Buddhist teacher Jack Kornfield advises, "We must find in ourselves a willingness to go into the dark, to feel the holes and deficiencies, the weakness, rage, or insecurity that we have walled off in ourselves. We must bring a deep attention to the stories we tell about these shadows, to see what is the underlying truth." When a lifetime of subconscious emotions surface, we face our evil twin, a stranger known in psychology as the shadow, the unwelcome visitor. We fear we *are* that stranger, wearing a mask yet also the mask itself. The work is to explore the vast territory that is us, and is also not us, over and over again. But each time, it becomes less frightening and stressful.

The Stress of Multiple Caregiving

For those who find themselves caregivers more than once, the cycle can seem unending. It is never easy, but the lessons carry over to make the next challenge easier to bear. In this way caregiving becomes a practice of devotion sanctified by repetition.

Anne, who is fifty-seven, calls herself a caregiver by nature and personality, having raised more than forty foster children with her husband over twenty years. She is also a caregiver by fate. After the death of her father-in-law, when she was in her thirties, she took care of her mother-in-law for two years in her own home. Her husband had melanoma surgery at age thirty-nine and passed away at fifty-eight from an aneurysm six months after he retired—and only two days after the death of her brother, who had a major stroke at forty-four and who also lived with Anne for two years, as his wife had left him. Then, two weeks after her husband died, Anne's mother, eighty-five, was diagnosed with ovarian cancer. And so she bought a little house next door and moved her parents in.

It was an unbelievable series of events. And yet taking care of her parents has changed Anne's life more than any of the others; she feels she has aged twenty years in the last four. She has gone on an antidepressant. She has witnessed both her mother and her father, married sixty-four years, become like small children. Her greatest stress is the fear of losing them—and the guilt about wanting this time to be over because the people she cares for are no longer the parents she knew. It grieves her to watch them watch each other's health decline. Her father, who is eighty-eight, has been gradually going downhill; his mind is weak and he has frequent transient ischemic attacks. Her mother has had several hospitalizations and bouts of chemotherapy, all of which erode Anne's stamina.

There hasn't been much time to assess the toll that caring for so many loved ones has taken. Anne's own dreams fell away when her husband died; they had just started to travel and had many wonderful plans. There have been times when she couldn't pray because of lost faith. Yet her five children and friends have carried her through periods of hopelessness. Although she had never been one to ask for help, proud to do things herself, stress has taught her to reach out.

I try desperately to be positive. I know in my heart and mind that I will get through this. I have also learned that people sincerely do want to help. Caregiving means you must be willing to give your all—I wouldn't have missed one foster child or the chance to take care of my parents for anything in the world. You need to adjust to loss even before the actual death. It never ceases to hurt more than you thought it would.

ACTION STEPS

Never ignore the pervasiveness of stress: it is often invisible and insidious. It is important to talk with other caregivers, to take time alone, to ask for help, and to learn to let go—of little things at first, just as a practice, to build confidence. It is equally important to get enough rest, exercise, and proper nutrition, and to laugh. It is all right to say no—you *can* set limits without closing your heart. Freeing up even a modicum of energy allows you to redeploy it for more heartfelt matters, acts that become regenerative rather than depleting.

In *Caregiver's Reprieve*, psychologist Avrene Brandt offers the following guidelines for coping with stress:

~ Identify the emotion. Fear, anger, guilt, depression—all have distinguishing features. Noting discomfort is a first step.

~ Admit the feelings exist and accept them as a part of being human.

~ Accept the emotion and distinguish between *having* it and *acting* on it.

~ Establish distance from the intensity of the situation, both physical and emotional, to moderate the feeling of being in constant turmoil.

~ Examine the reasons for your emotions, such as your thoughts, attitudes, and beliefs about how you are being treated.

~ Express your negative feelings—with the help of a mental health professional if needed. Dwelling on negative feelings by oneself can intensify and crystallize them.

~ Establish your identity beyond the role of caregiver by reaching out and relating to others.

Regret and guilt, anger and resentment: these are the offspring of caregiver stress. We have given them power, but we can also set them free. The truth is that love is stronger than fear. It is the heart that shows the vision of how life can be, even in the midst of suffering.

There is always hope: in the darkness lies the pathway out. As we enter the fearful places, we discover that it is we who dominate them, not the reverse. Meeting these unwanted emotions, acknowledging each of them, opens the way into a deeper truth, the substance of new life. At this stage we have more control than we think. We always have choice: the exhortation is to become aware that we do.

Blessings

In a dream, Dad is in the hospital, room 207; I'm in room 206. As I stand in the hallway, I notice he's reading *Hamlet*. I ask the significance and he replies, "Victory digs deep."

He announces he must leave. I know that, and thank him for my life. He assures me that everything that has happened is perfect, all of life is perfect. Then he simply ceases to exist, and I am caught up in an explosion of blinding, pearlescent light. I have no mass. I am just awareness, rocketing upward at warp speed. A thought materializes: "What about Mom?" And suddenly my father and I are back.

Something was shaking my bed as I hopscotched through dismal dreamscapes. Having arrived home in California only the night before, I clung to sleep; but as I became aware of a hand on my foot, I screamed. It was my husband, Bob, trying gently to awaken me. "Dad?" I asked, alarmed. He nodded; there had been a drug reaction, and Dad wasn't expected to make it.

Devoured at last, I disappeared between disbelief and panic. Nurse Nancy reported that my father had also contracted sepsis, a damning infection of the blood. Melanie also called, saying that Aunt Sam, who had once again tried her best, needed to leave as soon as a staff of caretakers could be put in place. For the first time I called my sister, Marcia, to ask for help, knowing it would be uncomfortable because she had not been close to our parents in more than twenty years. I was too exhausted to rush home. She insisted I not martyr myself; she would make the trip. I dreamed about my father all night, and waited for The Call.

It came the next morning. "Did you kiddos see *Calvin and Hobbes*?" Bob and I were agape: it was Dad, as if nothing had happened. He wanted to read the comic strip to us, and so we all laughed and Bob and I cried and didn't know what to make of life. Hesitantly, we asked how he was; he allowed that he was a mess and had dreamed he was in a hospital. "I almost got there," he told us, and we knew it was true.

Marcia set about reorganizing schedules; there were few choices. Both parents needed twenty-four-hour care, and no family member alone could provide it. The extreme option meant nursing home placement, so we took the middle route, combining home health and hospice workers for $3,700 a week. We donated our last funds to the outreach account; the next step would be Medicaid.

Even so, this careful system quickly became strained. Mother was gagging at every meal and had developed thrush, a persistent yeast infection on her tongue that had to be swabbed continually. My parents were on different sleeping and bathing and medication schedules. Mother wanted a warm home; Dad lay in pools of sweat. I had to go home again, so I decided to make it an occasion to honor my parents' forty-ninth wedding anniversary at the summer solstice—a celebration of love.

On my third day back, in walked Faye, lunch bag in hand and everything under control. A whirlwind of goodwill, she shook my father's hand, kissed my mother, and got down to business vacuuming and spot-cleaning. Sharp and fearless, she respected my parents and never treated them as invalids. Mother even allowed her complete range of the household. Best of all, Faye paid attention to her and made her laugh.

Faye and I accomplished so many projects, including cleaning out the garage so that I could move the office files there. Mother became obsessed with my project, incessantly prodding Dad to go look. The hospice aide and I were inexperienced, so transferring him into the wheelchair caused immediate pain. Knowing it was already a disaster but wanting to have done with it, Dad boiled and bumped and yelped down the narrow hallway, Mom hounding and hurrying him while I held the morphine pump and bladder bag. The footrest banged along the walls as he cursed and jerked the wheels just to get to the door some thirty feet away. He took a glance, agreed it was a great job, and hurried back to bed.

In those ten minutes he was totally spent, pain in every crevice while he bolused himself, but it was too late. He had forgotten the booster of morphine beforehand as insurance and was deluged by agony. Within ten minutes Mother was again persecuting him to see the garage, and he lashed out at her. Instantly he recoiled in shame and regret. Here was a man who had been keeping himself alive for a sweetheart who could no longer appreciate his sacrifice. From that moment Father never regained equilibrium; it marked the beginning of his last, long decrescendo.

The day I left, instead of her usual delay tactics, Mom softly led me over to Dad's bed, where she placed my free hand into his left hand and took his right hand so that we formed a circle. "I'm looking at the two most beautiful women in the world," he said as I leaned my head against my mother's.

My parents' illnesses had changed everything forever, exhaling me into oblivion to face the most horrible fears—and then breathing me back in again with blessings far greater than the losses. I begged to stay forever in our circle, to let this moment infuse all my days, yet knew it would slip away. But the love would last forever.

CHAPTER 8

Caregivers and Depression

It seems that we are humbled before the great events of life.
Events over which we have no power, no influence. Events
that do not play fair. To be humbled like this is not meant
to be punishment, but rather Death grooming us to awaken.
—Stephanie Ericsson, *Companion through the Darkness*

When we are so full of change and loss, when we have
ventured far from our comfortable cocoons into which
everything dear has been stored, sometimes we seem
trapped in a terrain that appears to offer nothing but anguish. Stream-
ing before us are icons of the life that used to be, the precious childhood and carefree youth that knew nothing of these adult torments.
We are lost in ourselves, in a sea of confusion. We feel alone, but what
we feel is not uncommon. Depression at midlife is both personal and
archetypal, writes licensed clinical psychologist Andrea Nelson in *Sacred
Sorrows*, "a headlong plunge into the deep unconscious where the self
confronts its disowned shadow in order to emerge empowered for the
role of wise elder."

One of the biggest health care crises, say doctors, psychologists, and social workers, is the depression faced by those who minister to aging relatives and friends—sometimes for decades. More than 60 percent of caregivers experience depression; the figure is higher among those who care for loved ones with dementia. Women in the general population suffer at twice the rate of men, with a fifth reporting clinical depression, which often requires medical intervention. It is double jeopardy: we anguish over what has happened to our loved one, as we are shaken by what is being required of us. We want to be good caregivers, but after a while we feel so inadequate and exhausted that we become unable to care at all.

It is time to understand that we cannot proceed until we take stock of our inner world, a crossroads that appears to threaten the very foundation of life. It is, as Carl Jung said, the dread and resistance over delving deeply into ourselves, the fear of the journey into hell. We may anesthetize and we may hustle, but that merely covers the feelings crying for attention.

Depression, however, may be inherent in our species. In *The Denial of Death*, cultural anthropologist Ernest Becker wrote that the fear of death haunts humanity like nothing else, pervading all activities. "The irony of man's condition is that the deepest need is to be free of the anxiety of death and annihilation, but it is life itself which awakens it, and so we must shrink from being fully alive."

Alzheimer's and Depression

Alzheimer's strikes a third to a half of people over eighty-five, mostly women. With this "oldest-old" population aging the fastest, the Alzheimer's Association projects that more than fourteen million North Americans now at midlife will contract the disease by 2050, unless cure or prevention is found. Globally, by the year 2025, thirty-four million are expected to contract the disease, with the greatest surge in developing countries. Not covered by most medical insurance because most patients need more supervisory than medical care, Alzheimer's disease can wipe out families: it is the third most expensive affliction after heart disease and cancer.

Alzheimer's caregivers are known as the hidden or second victims of the disease, as they commonly suffer from fatigue, stomach problems, headaches, sleeping difficulties, tension, anger, sadness, and especially depression. The cause is clear: because more than 70 percent of sufferers live at home, they are cared for by relatives and friends day and night over as many as twenty years. The typical caregiver for a relative with Alzheimer's spends an average of sixty-nine hours a week at it—many spend one hundred hours—and has been doing so for four years. Half live with their loved one. This is the proverbial "thirty-six-hour day."

In early stages, when words and short-term memories are slipping, caregivers are more optimistic—and uninformed—about the progression of the disease. But parallel to later, severe stages, where the loved one is manic and wandering, incontinent and sometimes expressing sad sexual behaviors, the care becomes more frustrating, the losses more irreversible.

According to recent studies, three-quarters of Alzheimer's caregivers are depressed at least occasionally, with a third who care for severe cases almost always depressed. They also experience a high rate of concurrent illnesses. With the help of family and friends, depression lessens; but community options to relieve this burden, such as specialized day care or assisted living, are not always available or affordable. Even so, one study found that when a loved one is in a nursing home or assisted-living facility, caregivers are more likely to be depressed than with their relative living at home. Caring and worrying go on unabated.

The tentacles of depression reach far and wide: into work and family dynamics, finances, and health. Emotions build on waves of disability, from powerlessness and unpredictability to loss of identity and lifestyle. As difficult behaviors—paranoia, combativeness, hallucinations—increase, caregivers work harder yet feel less able to manage them. It is hard to feel we are doing a good job when our loved one only continues to deteriorate. The disease becomes personal: rather than accepting it as a medical condition beyond the scope of a lay person to control, caregivers feel it is they themselves who are out of control and inadequate.

Sally cares for her mother, not her birth mother but the one who raised her. She works part time and has twins in college; her husband works two jobs to help with expenses. Her father cannot care for her mother, though he is free with criticism, so Sally brought her from the East Coast to live with her family in the Southwest. She says:

> Alzheimer's is filled with relief—knowing what is wrong—and simultaneous guilt, right from the start. Death only moves this into another stage, not helped by kindly strangers who never changed a diaper but now offer words of support you longed to hear through the many lonely hours. Hours and hours spent with a living being, someone you should know but no longer do, someone who might be better off dead than this breathing "thing" who stares vacantly. With Alzheimer's you grieve before the body dies, you grieve as you watch each little part go away, never to return.
>
> You lose yourself in this daily experience with death, and it becomes blurred in a line with your own life, much of which has died from lack of nutrition, of stimulation with the outside world. The world of the living, loving, working, laughing people never seems to find your door or your phone number, never sees you wither from lack of all human contact save that one who is a walking death before you. I can't remember anything but loneliness. I seem unable to reach out. I am so desperate for the touch of a hand, to be held. I go nowhere, I see no one. The world seems to want me to get over it and get on with it. There is no "it" for me to get on with.

Depression can come on gradually, but once it is entrenched, it is difficult to dislodge without help. It is critical that Alzheimer's caregivers seek education, respite, support groups, family interaction, hobbies, and social activities. It is also important to take care of legal and financial matters as soon as possible so that the loved one is still able to express his or her wishes and so that full attention and energy can be given to the person rather than to paperwork. Such legal matters include a durable power of attorney for health care, which authorizes someone to make decisions when the person becomes incapacitated, and a living will, which outlines preferences for end-of-life medical treatment.

Two notes: Because there is no rehabilitation possible, Alzheimer's disease (AD) does not qualify for Medicare insurance, which covers acute rather than chronic illness. However, if there is a concurrent condition such as a stroke, limited benefits may apply. It can be difficult to qualify for Medicare's hospice benefit because, although AD is a terminal illness, it is hard to assess when life expectancy will reach "less than six months," the federal regulation for admission to the program. In both cases, professional consultation is advised.

Clinical Depression

According to the National Mental Health Association, women suffer higher rates of clinical depression not just for biological reasons but also for social: they have greater stress from work and family responsibilities, roles and expectations, and poverty. Suppressing the normal grief that comes from sustained loss also can lead to chronic depression, which threatens both life and livelihood. Cultural values contribute layers of apprehension: "In a society that is defended against the tragic sense of life, depression will appear as an enemy, an unredeemable malady," writes philosopher Thomas Moore in *Care of the Soul*. There appears to be no direction but down—endless, sightless, meaningless. A loss of self is the result of pervasive disillusionment and alienation, the sense of having lost one's way even though at the time it seemed the only direction to go. When reactions to stress extend into feelings of worthlessness, that's depression, a signal that help is needed.

"We don't have a lot of self-worth and satisfaction from this role," says Suzanne Mintz, president and cofounder of the National Family Caregivers Association. "Satisfaction and pride are associated with a job well done, and we don't feel these things as much as we feel the difficult emotions." The greatest anxiety is that depression will never subside; there seems to be nothing to hold on to except that which dies. So family caregivers repress these unwelcome feelings—fatigue, hopelessness, guilt, irritability, emptiness—trying to do all things and fill all expectations, until there is nothing left but a hole where they used to be.

Breaking Down

It takes time to understand and break down emotional patterning; it takes time to survey the interior that has remained intimidating so much of our lives. Within us are countless specters of fear and loss, places we have shut away from the reservoirs of life. But only when these foreign chambers are entered can the spell be broken.

Judie charted the subtle emotional cycles over fifteen years of caring for her mother, Cornelia, who was a nurse in full awareness of what the diagnosis of Alzheimer's meant: in desolation, she called her daughter at all hours to insist she did not have AD.

Judie's initial period of helplessness ended after her sister gave her a T-shirt that read, "Just Do It!" She called the local Department of Aging, worked her way through social service agencies and elder care organizations, and amassed reading materials. She found support groups, adult day care, and visiting nurses and learned to ask for help instead of being resentful that no one was volunteering. Nothing was going to change despite her reaction to it, so she learned to live with it.

Judie, now fifty-seven, tried everything imaginable to provide the best care. She fired four of Cornelia's doctors because they would not give direct answers or felt they knew her mother better than she did after only one visit. Through connections at work she found a wonderful gerontologist, then a gerontology psychiatrist, and physical and occupational therapists. Her mother improved physically and in self-esteem; her neighbors kept watch and phoned if something seemed amiss. Then one day Judie made her usual call, and Cornelia took a long time answering. She said, "Something is wrong. I can't hold the phone. I fell down and now my hand won't work." Judie and her son rushed over and realized Cornelia had had a major stroke; half her body was paralyzed. After five weeks in the hospital Cornelia transferred to a rehabilitation unit, supposedly for five weeks. But after three, Judie was informed that Cornelia was as well as she was going to be, and Medicare would no longer cover her stay. Her mother was being summarily discharged.

That began the second leg of Judie's odyssey as primary caregiver, as her two siblings lived far away. She moved Cornelia into her home, canceling her ten-year-old's long-awaited sleep-over party, which made him feel less important than his grandmother. They kid-proofed the house again—throw rugs were taken up, a latch was installed high on the cellar door, caps were put on outlets, and the hot water temperature was lowered. Judie continued to work as a bank teller but had to cut back on her hours. She was passed over for promotions three times; her son was not adjusting to middle school well. She had no time for him and she knew it. Meanwhile her husband believed his mother-in-law was saying things just to annoy him. Judie's loyalties were being pulled in four directions at once. Everyone—husband, son, mother, job—wanted her full attention. She tried to comply.

Judie went from frazzled to frozen. Her son's grades fell, she and her husband fought constantly. She neglected her own health and abandoned church and friends. And so it continued until Cornelia became a danger to herself, trying to stuff garbage down the disposal or watering the night light instead of plants. Judie had never dealt with these kinds of problems before and had nothing to relate them to. She had no idea what she was doing, fearful she would accidentally kill her mother. When her husband hinted it was either Cornelia or him, Judie decided that having her mother at home was wrecking her family and found a personal care facility.

But the troubles didn't end there. She started hearing from Cornelia's siblings: "How dare you dump her in a home? Don't you love her enough to take proper care of her? What kind of daughter are you?" Judie finally told them she would sign over her power of attorney and they could take Cornelia home. No one offered. Still, she churned with guilt that she had not seen it coming sooner, that she could not do more, that she was ignoring her own family—guilt about the personal care and, later, guilt about the nursing home. One day she came home from work and could not stop crying. Two hours later her husband checked her into a psychiatric unit. Judie had a complete breakdown; she was there for just over a month.

It was actually a welcome turning point. "It was wonderful. I learned to set mental priorities, to be assertive without fear, to avoid 'peace-at-any-cost thinking,' and to cope with the problems of life." Between the support groups and her psychiatrist, she finally learned not to accept guilt placed on her by others. She learned the source of her anger and what to do about it. She was diagnosed with clinical depression and continues with Prozac and therapy.

In a way, Judie says, the hardest stage was acceptance: at first it felt more like giving up. It came by understanding that Cornelia was never going to get well and that she was not going to be able to care for Cornelia until she died. When her mother did pass away, after eight years in the nursing home, Judie was at peace and without regret. "You have to be able to give of yourself and put aside some of your personal goals and dreams and empathize with the care receiver. It was my faith and the grace of God that got me through this, so I vowed I would help anybody who found themselves in this situation." She has kept that promise.

The heartache and pressure of caring for people with mental illness can drive caregivers into clinical depression, one survey found. Women and nonworking caregivers are most at risk. Despite the many positive aspects of this work—the clear satisfaction in solving difficult problems, in developing maturity, and in keeping a loved one at home—these acts of love are time-consuming, labor intensive, and emotionally binding. Sometimes there are simply not enough physical, emotional, or financial resources to carry out our intentions. Being realistic means that we cannot always understand, predict, or control events. That does not mean we have failed.

Clinical depression—a low mood over a long period—is a costly medical illness, not only in terms of lost productivity and absenteeism from work but especially in reduced quality of life. It often goes untreated because people don't recognize the symptoms, such as withdrawal and sleeplessness, thinking these are normal for older people or during menopause, or because such depression is confused with grief. Denial, shame, and embarrassment also hamper resolution. Depression is highly treatable, however. It is not a sign of weakness or selfishness to take care of oneself; it is smart and necessary. If we burn out, there may be no one to take our place.

Compassion Fatigue

When caregiving becomes more stressful than satisfying, when sleep disturbances and an inability to leave the loved one become overwhelming, burnout ensues. One of the greatest sources of depression among caregivers is compassion fatigue—the inability over the long term to continue to draw forth the commitment and fulfillment of the early days. Studies have shown that the best predictor of institutionalization is the inability of the family to maintain the older person at home, rather than actual exacerbation of the medical condition. As people live longer and need more assistance, caregiver burnout is increasing: many people survive debilitating conditions that would have killed them years earlier and choose to live at home, which requires a twenty-four-hour family involvement.

One fifty-four-year-old woman has been caring for her husband for eighteen of their thirty married years; there is no end in sight. Four years ago he had a kidney transplant and they thought everything would be all right. But the medications are eating away his body, causing continual complications including bowel blockages, blood clots in his legs, and two surgeries to attach his feet to his ankles.

"The last eight years have been awful. I am the one who has to do the dirty work; my husband is too proud to let anybody but me wash him or take care of his needs. Illness is very controlling; and I think after a while love disappears and it's just duty. When our children were little, with their strollers and diapers, it was cute. To care for an ill person is not cute. It's just one thing after another."

And yet, love and duty abide, as in this story: "Today I, Anne, age fifty-one, am a caregiver, but no longer to my parents. I baby-sit with my childhood girlfriend's seven-month-old grandson. I'm doing this to get over what my husband, Carl, and I have gone through for the past five years as primary caregivers for my parents, Ruth and Bill, and as advocates for Carl's mother, Josephine."

Six years ago, Ruth was diagnosed with colon cancer; Bill was forgetting most recent events. Although Anne and her husband, two children, and two grandchildren lived a thousand miles away, primary duties fell to her. One day Bill couldn't find his car in the hospital parking lot after he visited Ruth. Anne called him at home and he said, "I'm exhausted. You'd better come here. I can't do this alone." When she got to California, he puzzled, "What are you doing here?"

And so it began, with total backing from Anne's family. Because Ruth was forgetting medications and other self-care tasks, Anne's objectives were getting her to quit a fifty-five-year smoking habit, giving her insulin injections, and taking care of continuous accidents with the colostomy bag. Not wanting to share a bedroom with her father, Anne exchanged the twin bed and dining room furniture and set up camp in the living room. Most nights she was summoned by one or the other parent. Ruth would have an accident trying to get to the bathroom, which meant comforting and changing her, then changing the bedding and washing shag carpeting and floors. Or Bill would fall getting out of bed—often into the dining room furniture—or just have anxieties, and she'd have to bandage him up or calm him down. She never got any rest, and the pressure started to build.

One day Anne borrowed her parents' car to get groceries. On the way, a man crashed into her. He was uninsured; she suffered from painful ribs. When she called home, she had to keep repeating the incident to her father. When her mother got on the phone she began screaming, "Now you've wrecked our brand-new car! What will we do?" Anne managed her way home only to find her parents frantic in the living room. "It's my seventy-fifth birthday and it's been absolutely the worst day possible!" her mother wailed, demanding cigarettes and throwing Anne's things around the room.

So Anne called her buddy Jan, for whose son she is now sitting, to take her away for the night. Bill begged her not to go. "I felt so sorry for him, but I was just too exhausted and hurt to continue. Boy, was I ever glad to see Jan drive up so I could get the heck out of there. I'd just deserted those two pitiful old frail people in their darkest hour, and I was elated."

But she felt guilty for leaving; they had done an excellent job of raising her. Even though they were treating her like a servant, this was how she was repaying them? She returned from her overnight respite with two bandaged ribs, determined to do everything she could; the love had not gone away, only a portion of herself. Anne was desperate to return to her own family, but Ruth insisted she stay, threatening to leave their money to any hired housekeeper. "All the money you have in the world isn't worth being away from my husband and my own home," Anne cried. But of course she stayed.

Incredibly, the next morning a home care agency's flyer was left on her front porch offering housework, medication supervision, meal preparation, and personal services. Anne called; Candy was a godsend. Ruth liked her, and Anne thought they had it made. After five months she left for Colorado, thirty-seven pounds lighter and feeling free.

But it was not the end. Over the next several months she spoke often with her parents; things were never going well. Then one day Ruth's doctor called, announcing that the cancer had spread. He didn't expect her to live long and insisted Anne come back at once. She and Carl cried a lot about it, but still she dropped everything and went straight to the hospital, finding her mother in restraints because she had been getting out of bed and falling, yelling for help so loudly that the nurses moved her as far from their station as possible. Anne knew she had to get her out of there.

It was time for a nursing home, so Anne searched out the best one. When Ruth found out, she sighed, "So I'm dying." All Anne could do was nod and cry. Carl came to visit. A week later Ruth died, at seventy-five. The home aide stayed on for Bill, and the couple returned to Colorado. Two months later Carl's mother passed away after a fall in a nursing home. The following month, their daughter married a financial whiz who convinced them to move to California to live with Bill, who by then had emphysema and Alzheimer's and was deaf. After a year and a half, continually asking when Ruth was coming home, he passed away at age eighty, not remembering who Anne was but referring to her sometimes as "the woman of the house." She still thought he was the sweetest man in the world.

Through all the things she did for her parents—taking care of her mother's flower beds, reading to her father, playing classical music and Trivial Pursuit—Anne hopes she has set a good example for her children. "My mother once told me when a dear friend died, 'Nothing is worse than trying to keep someone alive and having them die anyhow.' It's true. It leaves the greatest hole in you. But even if the kids don't benefit, we have the satisfaction of knowing we did all we could for our parents. The heart of caregiving means loving some people in this world enough to give up your life for them."

Beyond the physical reasons, however, are deeper causes for caregiver burnout and depression, notes spiritual teacher Ram Dass. These include expectations of specific results, self-doubt as to whether you're up to the tasks and blame if you are not, and the difficulty of setting limits without feeling guilty. It's not always our efforts that burn us out, he writes in *How Can I Help?*, but where the mind stands in relation to them. The problem of burnout is not the work itself but how much self-importance we invest in it.

Ram Dass explains that the more we take credit or place blame, the more we burn out. We become so identified with our roles that we believe we wield influence beyond true measure. Instead, he proposes a shift of perspective to that of the witness, who works in cooperation with life forces over which we have no control, a player among them. When it is no longer our identity and self-esteem that are at stake, our focus comes off ourselves to the activities at hand. We learn to be present in the moment but not lost in the part we play.

Suicide: Feeling There Is No Other Way Out

At the extreme margins, a caregiver can become so consumed by duty, so running on empty, that her own life is on the line. Here, the decision to take charge is literally one of life and death. Jo has survived the worst consequences of more than seven ragged years of depression and sleeplessness. She became a caregiver to her mother in her own older age. Already somewhat frail, having had surgery several times and maintaining a house and home business, she juggled all her duties alone. She couldn't afford a housekeeper, and her family lived away.

Living with her mother, Jo tended to the ever-increasing demands of a dementing illness coupled with hearing loss. She didn't know about Medicaid at the time, and there wasn't much day care available because Alzheimer's patients weren't accepted in those days. Her mother was a night wanderer and kept wanting to walk home—to Germany. Several times Jo had to call the police. Her mother didn't sleep at night, so Jo didn't either. She put locks everywhere, and gated the top of the stairs; but one morning at two o'clock, she found her mother ready to climb over the banister.

Jo grew haggard; she hurt financially as well because she had abandoned her business to care for her mother. She vividly remembers the breaking point: It was a hot August night. The windows were wide open, and she worried that her mother would wake the neighbors with her foghorn voice. "Something was upsetting her. She insisted on going downstairs and I pushed her toward her bedroom, trying to shush her. She resisted and started hollering. Finally I managed to get her to bed, and she was shouting that she wanted to go home. I was pulling the covers over her and she was shouting and I saw the pillow next to her— I tend to visualize all kinds of scenes—and I knew how someone could easily put the pillow over her mouth."

But Jo could never do that. Instead, "the only way out that I thought of was to kill myself. I went into my room and tried a plastic bag—it hurts, believe me." Her mother quieted down, perhaps frightened by the expression on her daughter's face. Jo says she wanted to die right there, so untenable had life become. Yet she had enough presence to call the police and the Alzheimer's Association hot line. At four o'clock in the morning, a wonderful volunteer asked what was the matter. Jo couldn't answer; hysterical, she burst out crying.

The next morning the Department of Aging phoned, Jo's call having been traced. They calmed her down and said help was coming, the first time anyone had offered. They had her mother evaluated at a psychiatric hospital, where she remained for three weeks, which allowed Jo some respite—and probably saved her life. She told the authorities then that she needed help at home, but because of her suicide attempt, her mother was not allowed to return. So Jo picked out a convalescent home, and her mother loved it. She had friends and a social life. For one of them, life was restored.

Jo, however, was not out of the woods; she almost died of peritonitis. "Caregivers are victims too. I did take care of her, I did risk my life, I ended up in poverty. What more could a daughter do?" Her mother passed away almost five years later; today Jo is an outspoken advocate for caregivers.

Suicide is the most dramatic expression of self-isolation and the eighth leading cause of death in North America. Rates increase with age and are highest among people sixty-five and older, especially the divorced or widowed. Those at highest risk experience great loss, ill health, and depressive illness—traits commonly found in the caregiving orbit.

And yet if the loss is shattering enough, the disillusionment deep enough, the call is heard from within, says clinical psychologist Connie Zweig. Some may refuse to respond. Those who listen will enter a dark but holy place, a symbolic death of the old ways. New life is poured from this depth.

ACTION STEPS

To cope with the effects of long-term caregiving and to mitigate the possibility of depression, professionals offer the following tips:

~ Have your loved one's problems diagnosed as early as possible to know what you're up against. Bring a list of questions and don't leave until you have the answers.

~ Educate yourself about the disease or condition from which your loved one suffers. Use national organizations, books, professionals, and the Internet.

~ Do legal and financial planning to protect assets before a crisis hits. Being proactive rather than reactive puts more control in your hands.

~ Know what community resources are available by calling your local department of aging. Ask for brochures and other helpful literature. Don't allow superstitious fears to prevent you from seeking information early. You cannot hasten a loved one's demise by preparing for eventualities.

~ Seek psychiatric or support group help if you feel overwhelmed or cannot stop dwelling on negatives. Ask for help from family, neighbors, and friends.

~ Take breaks, both long and short. It is important to relax whenever possible.

~ Maintain activities that you enjoy; don't assume you have to give up everything. This is about love, not martyrdom.

~ Learn the symptoms of stress and depression, such as blurred vision, digestive problems, high blood pressure, excessive drinking, headaches, lack of concentration, and loss of appetite.

~ Don't dwell in regret or wallow in "if only."

~ Be realistic, keep a sense of humor, and don't forget to breathe.

Depending on our response to intense caregiving, we can contract hypertension, cardiac problems, weight gain, bad backs, ulcers, and a host of immune-deficient illnesses. These are the physical manifestations of depression; and yet, even when they are controlled, we remain unsettled.

Loss of heart is almost a disease in itself: defeat, disillusionment, a crumbling of stable reference points. When we believe in the absolute fixedness of our values and opinions, when we expect perfect solutions, facing the illness and ultimate death of a loved one can rip open our neat philosophical packages, leaving a void where meaning used to be.

Life involves change and change involves pain. Sometimes the pain is unbearable, and we run from it in haste. Abandoning it, however, we also quit on ourselves and lose the potential for transcending it. In a soulful sense, the desperation that leads to depression is also a cry for transformation. It may seem unlikely that good could come out of so much pain. But it is possible: something needs to die so that another, deeper something may live.

Depression, says Thomas Moore, is a rite of passage to higher levels of self-realization. It is a process of the aging of the soul, no longer clinging to the ideals and qualities of youth but looking to the wisdom of experience. In newfound self-acceptance and self-knowledge there is a "halo of melancholy" but also a peace impossible in earlier years. He suggests that depression is initiation into the catharsis of emptiness, the dark places where the soul also resides. Depression even might carry its own angel who guides us to special insight and vision.

It is an almost instinctual act of self-preservation: we are about to be annihilated by change, but we are not yet ready, not able, to let the unknown take over. Just as adrenaline protects us at the physical level, profound depression can be a mechanism for slowing us down and making us pay attention. If we accept inner torment as a directive toward wholeness, we will climb out of the valley of the shadow of death with restored life. The proposition is to explore this self-scape so that we may defuse any harm.

We must never underestimate the power of depression to rocket us far from well-being. We must also never underestimate the might of our inner resources to carry us back home. They rise from our depths: feelings of worthlessness, apathy, sadness, helplessness, and thoughts of death or suicide are all messages of fragmentation demanding attention. "A life lived afraid of our shadows is only half a life, driven by the constant necessity to prove to ourselves, to our mothers, or to the culture, that we are some sort of ideal selves, instead of fully ourselves," writes Jungian analyst Naomi Ruth Lowinsky in *Stories from the Motherline*.

In this journey that dissociates us from former relationships and identities, we can feel absolutely schizophrenic. But in the depths of anguish simmers a new kind of faith. Michael Washburn offers hope in the face of hopelessness: "Despair is not an utterly negative condition. It is a condition astir with positive possibilities. For the process of dying to the world that leads to despair stimulates a yearning for life that, unbeknownst to the despairing person, draws on hidden spiritual resources."

In this outpost of solitude our faith is tested to the extreme, for it is only when we hit bottom that we can see another direction, one that opens into a larger world filled with something other than ourselves.

CHAPTER 9

Hitting Bottom

Deep in the wintry parts of our minds, we are hardy stock and know there is no such thing as work-free transformation. We know that we will have to burn to the ground in one way or another, and then sit right in the ashes of who we once thought we were and go on from there.—Clarissa Pinkola-Estés, *Women Who Run with the Wolves*

Caregivers often wonder at the pale discomfort that haunts their sleep, the unresolved naggings that remain secluded in psyche and spirit. These are voices that will no longer be denied, for it is here that a new, even more intense battle takes shape. It is on this field that spirit announces itself. This is a critical stage on the caregiving journey, for it is the point at which we have been stretched to the maximum. We have hit bottom, the farthest extent of who we thought ourselves to be. There seem to be only two choices: snap back to where we started or break apart entirely.

But there is another path. Carl Jung defined the attainment of any extreme position at which it begins to turn into its opposite as the *enantiodromia*. This is a legendary event as in the story of Inanna, the Sumerian Queen of Heaven and Earth, and her sister goddess Ereshkigal, Queen of the Underworld. This myth describes Inanna's journey to visit her sick sister. It is not an easy descent; Inanna suffers loss after loss of prestige and power, of emotional certainty and lifestyle. This stripping away is the price paid for reaching "the depths within ourselves that we otherwise might not reach," says Jean Shinoda Bolen. These depths reveal soul issues, a merging of beauty and beast.

On successive turns in the labyrinth, it is at each lowest point where a shift takes place. If we let ourselves go all the way in and touch bottom, something magical happens: just as becoming a caregiver has entailed taking a path that reversed the direction of our life, so does another path open up at a certain stage of growth. At the summit of crisis, inner powers appear. A voice beckons, and it is time to leave the old life.

Crisis becomes the call from the higher self to meet the unlived life, to resurrect those dormant powers that yearn to live. As illustrated in Dante's famous descent to inferno, at the nadir of his journey when he identifies and confronts the Shadow, he is carried past this beast and discovers who rules the soul. Our best meets our worst and finds harmony; separation is illusion.

Life more abundant begins when one finds the only possible course is back outward—but not to turn one's back on the journey inward. Reduced by apparent loss, we have become humble enough to live in the moment. At this turning point of no return, we are swallowed up by what we have most feared and are alchemized into more than we were. A doorway opens into another way of being, one wide enough to encompass every experience. Living at our center we see all directions, releasing the self-indulgent version of life. We glimpse the infinity of being, spread out before us: no longer is there a need to preserve the ideal at the expense of our true nature.

"We cannot let go of anything we do not accept," says meditation teacher Stephen Levine. "The fear which has always guarded these heavy emotions from exploration now becomes an object of examination and acts as a guide into new territory. Fear becomes an ally which whispers that we are coming to our edge, to unplumbed depths, to the space in which all growth occurs."

This juncture between past and future frames the remainder of the caregiving experience—and the rest of life. In myth, Elysium is the underworld place where hardships occur, but not without the gift of meaning and learning. It is the reflection of the topside world where everything is seen as gain or loss. Down below, everything is interpreted through the development of inner strength and knowing. Down below, the shadow becomes the beacon, lighting the way. Down below, we become both beacon and light and guide our own way home.

To the Stars through Difficulty

In a dream, I'm at Bard College, my father's alma mater, near
a river in New York City, strolling along beautiful paths lined
with trees and statues. At one end of the long parkway is a
filigree gate. I enter and am back in Wichita, in the rear seat
of a car Dad is driving, with Mom in the front and my deceased grandmother to my right. He is heading to the airport indirectly, past his high school and other youthful land-
marks. Grandma is impatient with her son's delay, but I am
looking beyond her to a gleaming colonial-style building
with a long passageway of pillars and immense columnar
trees, an ethereal golden-auburn light resplendent from far
beyond. I realize that Father wants to visit these memories
before he leaves. Grace descends as I understand that he is
not finished with his life review, giving me a peace I never
thought possible.

I was dancing the agony and the ecstasy on the head of a pin. I
had no will of my own; the "I" that was . . . was no longer me. A
new me was becoming, but not yet born. A still, small voice kept
repeating: anyone who follows her heart cannot fail. And so I
continued on.

All summer Dad was less available by phone; he even chastised
me once, saying he didn't have time to chitchat. I knew it was the
morphine, but it cut to the bone. Mother began falling frequently,
three times in five days, skinning her knees crawling to the door for
help. When she tripped and hit her head and hip near Dad, he
cried, straining helplessly as sirens rushed her to the hospital. Aunt
Sam hurried back to town, but when she saw her sister-in-law lying
there so small and helpless, she realized she could not stay at all.
She returned home directly, pulverized by her inability to visit her
brother and worried that she might actually be the next to die.

How I wanted to avoid the cruelest decision, but I no longer
could. Mother's insistence on using the stairs was a safety hazard;

home aides were forbidden to carry her up and down any longer, even with a belt. The health agency threatened to pull out altogether: Dad was refusing to allow overnight aides to have any lights on, or monitors, insisting they sit, immobile, in his darkened room all night long. Mother refused to sleep in a second hospital bed next to Dad; she wanted familiar privacy upstairs.

In their desperation to retain control, my parents had become dangers to themselves. With my consent, social workers found a newly refurbished room in a nursing facility about two miles from the condo. To reserve it, we needed to complete the paperwork at once. We assumed Dad would never agree, but when he was told there was only enough money to keep them at home for a month, he relented. Incredibly, at the same time a reporter from the *Wichita Eagle*, where Dad was assignments editor in the 1940s, called about writing an article on my parents to help raise funds. I knew my father would be horrified, yet it was our last hope. I told him up front; he was concerned people would think less of them. I argued that was impossible; the community would want to give back.

In our dimmest hour civic support lifted us up. All segments responded—educational, political, religious, business, and medical— as well as fraternal clubs, Mother's music sorority and hairdresser, and former neighbors. Yet even though our prayers had been answered, the sparkle in Dad's voice had slipped into resignation. He hated taking what he felt was charity; he hated feeling weak.

Four days after my father's seventieth birthday, my parents left their home in the glory of a summer Kansas day, the thrumming of cicadas against a radiant scent of loam and hay. Again asking the paramedics to pause, Father breathed in the earth and felt the sun's warmth as Mother went ahead with an aide. Only fifteen minutes before they left, she was informed they were going somewhere they could get straightened out. She never had a chance to take in what was happening, to say good-bye to her Steinway or her memories. All the possessions they held dear, the familiar surroundings, the contributions that reflected their hard work, all were left behind for safety and for finances. They traded their past for a dreary future, one without hope, privacy, or pleasure.

Once settled in their room, decorated by some of their personal effects now labeled against theft, Mother bore into the aide and cackled almost unintelligibly, "I want you out of here right after dinner. We don't need you. We don't want you!" She weighed only seventy pounds, but her words struck with brute force.

PART III

Bridges to
the Future

CHAPTER 10

Support Strategies and Everyday Miracles

We have not even to risk the adventure alone, for the heroes of all time have gone before us; the labyrinth is thoroughly known; we have only to follow the thread of the hero-path.—Joseph Campbell, *The Hero with a Thousand Faces*

W e are not alone. We are never truly alone. In the contours between the old life and the new, there are signposts that connect the journey. These bridges come in all forms and at every plane of existence, from physical to spiritual. They are the friends who comfort us or give respite, the leaps of faith made solid, the everyday miracles that pull us out of despair. There are supports everywhere, waiting to be recognized and accepted.

Dealing with issues at the end of life, however, caregivers feel very alone. Decisions about life support and questions about the meaning of suffering permeate the everyday tasks and bring caregivers to a new threshold. They become members of the invisible fellowship of those who bear the mark of pain, as Albert Schweitzer called those who know anguish but find friendship in common wounds. It is magical to discover, one-on-one or in a group, that others understand. That knowledge alone can carry us over troubled waters. It also can mean the difference between dysfunction and coping, for commonalty frees us from the desolation we fear only we have known.

Traditional Family and Cultural Supports

We want to believe there is an identifiable solution to every problem, that all we need is to hook up to some toll-free number. Yet what caregivers need most are support and validation, and the best source is others who can empathize. We heal by sharing experiences, which builds a bridge for all who follow. Caregiving becomes a rite of passage, a redemptive crossroads to larger life.

Quality of life is the bottom line in caregiving, but it cannot exist in a vacuum. Family bonds are essential to the wellness of all concerned, and are the first line of defense in the battle against loneliness and frustration. Despite suggestions to the contrary, there is good news: Donna Wagner, director of gerontology at Towson University in Maryland, observes that even though outside help may be needed with long-term care, "the evidence is not so much that we have a social problem, but that we have a tenacious and flexible family structure that works no matter what."

Need can draw out the best in families. "Caregiving has really just become my way of life," says Ameta, forty-four, who can barely remember when her mother, Callie, took care of her. Ten years ago Callie had an aneurysm, which hospitalized her for three months; at the same time, Ameta's father had leukemia. She went to her parents' home every day to cook meals, give medicines, and help with her mother's physical therapy. Then a year later Callie had a hip replacement because of osteoporosis and was in a wheelchair. One Sunday Ameta went by on her way to church to give them some medicines. "Dad was sitting in his recliner asleep, never to wake up again on this earth. This is when it all really began."

Blessed with an unusual capacity for loyalty, Ameta's fifteen-year-old son moved in to take care of his grandmother while Ameta couldn't be there; a year later she and her twelve-year-old daughter moved in as well. What they didn't know was that the aneurysm was a prelude to Alzheimer's. Ameta was still trying to make Callie do everything right, correcting her constantly and upsetting her. Still, Ameta and her children became a natural caregiving team: Ameta's son even fixed his grandmother's hair for church as well as she did.

Ameta has been grateful for the opportunity to take care of Callie, whom she cherishes. A few years ago Ameta remarried; they moved a short distance away. She visited at least three times a day to take care of everything and had Meals on Wheels deliver lunch daily. Her mother still phoned three dozen times a day, having lost all sense of time. A year ago, Callie became combative and inconti-nent, was falling a lot, and had to be lifted and changed. Even so, Ameta's son and his new wife wanted to move in and take care of Callie, as did her daughter and new son-in-law. Ameta's new husband wanted Callie to move in with them. But she had to be placed in a nursing home, where she climbed over the bed rail and fell, breaking her hip into four pieces. She also has had several strokes and her vi-sion is declining.

Yet she knows Ameta's voice. Some days she is sweet, some days cranky and blaming every bad thing on her daughter. But if Ameta starts to sing an old gospel song, Callie doesn't miss a word. She can still quote scripture and say full prayers. "My husband says that is because that's where her spirit is, even though her mind may be messed up. You have to just love them with all your heart, be as patient as you can, and take it a step at a time."

Although every culture places value on taking care of elders, their means may be submerged by the mainstream. Some cultures main-tain their family traditions more than others. For example, among African Americans in the past, says Dr. Peggye Dilworth-Anderson, professor of human development and family studies at the University of North Carolina at Greensboro, there was one primary caregiver in most families. "But in families where you have increased poverty, eco-nomic uncertainty, and multiple needy generations instead of one, we may see multiple primaries. In the historical development of the black family, during times when it looked like they were not going to make it, they did, because of adaptive strategies. Everyone looked out for each other. The culture had enough flexibility that kin and nonkin could serve in caregiving roles." Even though today black women suffer more than the general population from poor health and finances, Dilworth-Anderson's research has found that black caregivers tend to experience fewer feelings of burden and depression: one positive outcome of caregiving is the value of filial piety, the need to support the elderly. "When people can do for their parents the way they should, it's an uplifting experience. If you adhere to the traditional ideology—and parent care is traditional—the ability to do that raises a person's sense of well-being."

Support Groups

In primitive societies, there were mourning rituals and social supports that helped restore harmony to both the individual and the tribe. In modern times, despite cultural differences, we increasingly turn in our grief and anxiety to groups grown not out of tradition but out of immediacy. In the past twenty years, self-help has flourished as people search for connection and resolution. When friends abandon us out of fear of contagion or because they haven't the capacity to hold another's suffering, we look for others with similar fears and hopes. We want to know that we are real, that what we are doing matters. Sharing stories becomes a modern-day ritual, with all the wisdom and solace of ancient lore. Something profoundly surprising also happens: when strangers reach out to strangers, they create family.

Caregivers actually rely less on health care professionals for coping strategies than on informal networks, including religious congregations. Today, sponsored by hospitals, social service agencies, and health associations, there are groups for most medical conditions, havens for resources, referrals, and restitution for a mobile society whose family and community links know more uprooting than grounding. "The fact that these groups are mushrooming . . . in itself is a clue about the magnitude of difficulties that families and patients face with illnesses that entail long-term declines," writes Marilyn Webb in *The Good Death*.

For many, these circles of support are simply a place to begin questioning. "People first come to groups looking for answers, to solutions for their problems," says Rich, who, while he was caring for his mother, attended a flurry of them and now leads one weekly. "After a while, though, the reason for the support group is the *support*.

We don't have pat answers because each case is unique, but we help people take the road that works for them."

Rich says the sessions are a safe place to explore feelings. At first the groups gave him back laughter, a precious commodity he had all but lost in the illogic and frustration of crises. He felt like Sisyphus, endlessly pushing a boulder up a hill. But Rich discovered that within those labors something more enduring was being accomplished: a chance to contemplate what his parents gave him. Listening to the troubles of group members has convinced him that society does not value the elderly—the older you get, it seems, the less you count. "Caring for a parent is not something you would ever wish on anybody, but we all have something in us of that universal love. You get this opportunity to do things for them, and while you're doing them it's hell for you because it's a total disruption in your life. And then you realize that's what life is all about, this helping. There isn't anything else."

Doctors, social workers, psychologists can't be all things to all people all the time. Sharing your feelings, venting outrage with others who will not criticize but instead help you move forward, grows a sense of closeness few professional relationships can equal. From this consolation more confident and intelligent care flows forth to the loved one. And the attention is returned to the caregiver in even greater measure because we discover we are not alone.

Professional Support

Until recent times, an increasingly frail elder had two options: to remain at home with family or to go into a hospital or nursing home. In response to a mushrooming demand for pragmatic family supports, there has been prodigious growth in such new industries as adult day care, hospice, elder law, assisted-living housing, care management counseling, workplace elder care benefits, and home health care. There are also psychiatric social workers, dietitians, podiatrists, continence advisers, physical therapists, and wound nurses who commonly interact with caregivers. Today it is not only about choices; it is also about honoring life. So when family reinforcements aren't available, the professionals provide surrogate support.

Robert's mother, Elvira, married at age sixteen. Because there was only one set of relatives she was close to, the stage was set for isolation after her husband passed away twenty years ago. She continued to work as a graphic artist but didn't drive, so Robert became chauffeur. After retiring, she spent her days window shopping with her sister, getting her hair styled every week, maintaining her finances and home. More than ten years ago, however, Robert noticed some subtle but persistent oddities, such as wanting him to oversee her checking account and throwing keys at bank personnel because she didn't want her safety deposit box anymore. He took her to a hospital for a geriatric evaluation, upon which she was diagnosed with advanced dementia. She was sixty-eight; Robert was forty-seven.

Even though he worked full time and was married, Robert visited his mother daily, fed the dog, and took care of bills. One time he found Elvira crying over the mail, saying, "I'm getting worse, I'm getting worse." Everything seemed to be spiraling out of control until a hospital geriatrician visited and made suggestions to improve the safety of her home, like a holding bar in the shower bathtub. Robert met with her weekly to discuss which agencies offered custodial home care and to validate his concerns. These talks started him on the right track, which has continued to this day in the form of smart counsel from caring professionals.

In order to protect his mother's assets, Robert sought conservatorship. He also hired trained caregivers for custodial care. Yet the aggravations continued. One day Elvira tried to push an aide down the stairs. Then there was combativeness, incontinence, and feces around the house. Time came for Robert to place her in a nursing home nearby, for $4,000 a month. On the attorney's advice, Robert sold his mother's home and put her cash assets into annuities and certificates of deposit. Even though this arrangement has entailed a lot of record-keeping and reporting, he believes the advice has helped keep Elvira comfortable and prolong her life.

For all of Robert's attentive care, however, his stress built up to near explosion. He fell prey to muscle spasms around the heart and severe tension headaches; then his union went on strike. His doctor put him on tranquilizers to control anxiety because he felt he was deteriorating along with his mother.

What brought me back from this ordeal is the fact that I was in constant communication with the professionals. I didn't try anything on my own. Once I knew what I was dealing with, I accumulated as much information as possible—reading, a group therapy session. It's been stressful and time-consuming, but the experience I have in this field—financial, medical, and legal—is an accomplishment. I know whom to call, where to go, what questions to ask. What causes more stress, though, is that when she passes on, it's forever. I made sure I told her I loved her before and after she became ill. My mom made me realize to take my life seriously—don't waste a minute. Smart lady.

Day Care and Care Management

Adult day care centers are becoming one of the most popular forms of support for caregiving families. For an average of $50 a day, they offer health and therapeutic services and social activities for people with functional or cognitive impairments and keep many elders living in the community instead of being institutionalized.

"Day care makes a lot of things possible," says one caregiver with two toddlers. "Otherwise I wouldn't have any options. I couldn't go to work and I would have to put Mother in a home. And at the center the staff reinforces their clients' dignity. They make them feel they're still a part of society. It's so important that people really understand that."

One of a new breed of aging network professionals is the care manager, usually a social worker or nurse who helps a family make and monitor a flexible plan of care. For a fee of $65 to $350 for the initial assessment—then subsequent hourly rates ranging from $30 to $150 depending on duties, credentials, and geographic location—professionals provide a range of services including in-home geriatric assessment, financial management, arranging for in-home care or long-term placement, and developing and monitoring a care schedule.

Rebecca's eighty-eight-year-old mother lives on the opposite coast, where she maintained an active life for many years after her husband died. Then her friends began to die, and she had difficulty paying bills and managing a household because her memory was faltering.

Rebecca, fifty-three and a family therapist, debated whether to bring her mother three thousand miles to live with her family or to place her in an assisted-living facility in her own community, where she would have her own apartment but also supportive services. Her mother insisted on independence, but she became depressed after her other daughter died. Rebecca called her husband's employee assistance program's information-and-referral number and found a care management organization to assess her mother's situation. Together they created a plan including Meals on Wheels, transportation to doctors, and periodic reassessments.

It's made a huge difference, Rebecca believes, both in her mother's well-being and in reducing the guilt over not doing the caregiving herself. Most of all, her mother now has companionship, which can prevent a host of serious complications related to isolation and depression. "For the first time I feel I have support with experts in aging, people knowledgeable about resources in her community. They do things my mother wouldn't let me do, but somehow with all of us working together, she will accept the services. I felt like I should know more; I was totally lost trying to go back there and set up services. I feel this is in her best interest, and it takes so much burden off. It's respectful of what she wants."

It cannot be emphasized enough: *We are not alone.* There are networks of formal and informal support available at all levels of need. Some are for the care receiver, some specifically for the caregiver. Any help at all, however, will always benefit the entire family. Support saves lives.

The Internet

One of the newest forms of social support is the World Wide Web, which has turned the Internet into virtual communities. This palpable network allows family caregivers to find companionship at all hours, a link to sanity through bulletin board forums, e-mail lists, databases, and live chats. People seek information for medical concerns, local resources, and services, but most of all they tap into the wellspring of experience. And they do it from the anonymity of their homes, often after putting a parent to bed or alongside a bedridden spouse.

Although computer work can be solitary, this technological forum brings together diverse people from all over the globe who share both suffering and solutions. It is an unprecedented equalizer: there are no economic or ethnic barriers, no geographical provincialism, no ageism or gender bias. The Net allows people to take charge of their lives and then extend a hand to others.

Says one chat group member:

> Something magical happens when people who share similar situations get together, as in a support group on-line. You may have a lot of questions, you may want more information. Since everyone in the group has been there or is there now, there is a sense of trust. Maybe there is a creative way of handling a problem you hadn't thought of or a way to find humor after a terrible day. Sharing your feelings with your loved one is not always possible anymore, but on-line, heads nod with understanding as you speak. Here you feel relief, the release of pent-up tension that comes with knowing your emotions are not so different.

Personal outpourings are welcome. It isn't spelling or speed that counts, but human contact. For Werner of Munich, Germany, a U.S.-based Alzheimer's e-mail list has been a lifeline, connecting him with caregivers in Israel, Australia, Great Britain, and New Zealand. Public attention for Alzheimer's disease (AD) is very limited in Germany, he says. The Web has become an adoptive community, taking him through a major life transition. Before his mother developed AD, Werner lived his own life. He worked in Stuttgart for two years, in Italy for four. Now, however, the disease rules his life. "I have never felt a continuous stress like I am feeling for three years. The moments I can live for myself are many times precious; most of the time my emotions go to my mother."

Werner is able to send his mother to day care, which provides needed respite, but he finds their greatest soothing in music. Brahms' "Alt-Rhapsodie" is the ultimate. Without it, he feels he could not survive. Werner shares his love of music with his Web friends. In return, he has learned invaluable coping skills, not only in recognizing stages of the disease, but also for self-improvement. "I was rather a great egoist. I did not do bad things to my mother, but sometimes I could have done better: I ignored the first stages of AD. If you flee from responsibility, you will be punished by yourself. Our subconscious knows very well when we did not try our best. And one day the unresolved life tasks come back and want to be resolved. Do it better now."

On-line relationships can become the strongest in a caregiver's life. There are no judgments, no masks, and no social obligations. Betty's friendships have buoyed her through isolating times. She vows she has never met such good friends as she has since going on-line. She never knew she would need them all so much. She went through months of caring for her argumentative mother-in-law and sick husband, both of whom lived at home and didn't get along. Marc suffered from heart problems after a stroke, as well as high blood pressure and kidney cancer. One day when he complained of excruciating pain in his left arm, Betty had to determine who needed help more. They decided to place his mother in a nursing home because the tension had contributed to Marc's mild heart attack.

Betty says her on-line support groups feel like family, because most of her relatives live far away or are not communicative. She had quit work to be with Marc in his retirement, thinking she could handle two housebound people. She struggled to find a nursing home and to get her mother-in-law on Medicaid; then doctors discovered that Marc had double renal failure. Both kidneys were recently removed—after other surgery for a tumor on his esophagus—and he is on dialysis. The couple has great confidence that his health will improve now. Through it all, her Internet friends have been a lifeline: she believes their prayers worked, and her gratitude is boundless. "These wonderful chat rooms have made such a difference. What else in life is there but to care about others?"

ACTION STEPS

~ Become familiar with the range of health care professionals who handle the problems of older people, such as geriatricians, home health aides, and social workers.

~ Investigate community and professional resources and support systems, including assistive or shared housing, adult day care, respite, hospice care, elder law, care management, and financial planners. They exist to serve consumers in need.

~ Set up informal support networks to monitor your loved one, often through a community's "gatekeeper" program, which ties in to local social services. These gatekeepers include postal workers, bank tellers, grocery store clerks, newspaper delivery people, utility readers, pharmacists, apartment managers, and bus or van drivers. Talk to neighbors whenever possible. "Telephone reassurance" is a service provided in many communities; volunteers phone daily to check on your loved one. Look into local volunteer companion and visitation services.

~ Using the Internet, support groups, or books and articles, familiarize yourself with the range of international services and information available about medical conditions, social services, financial aid, and legal and housing options. Regular common-sense precautions also apply here.

~ Be aware of the hidden demands and expectations placed on adults by society and culture that contribute to a sense of isolation and guilt.

~ Don't feel you have to stick with one solution if it isn't working out. Be flexible and pay attention.

Alternative Health Care

Especially in an era of rationed health services, where it is feared that the effort to save money means withholding appropriate care, people yearn for a more humanistic approach. Traditional medicine has set its sights on diagnosis, treatment, and cure of physical systems: drugs and surgery. But gaining popularity are alternative, integrative, and complementary medicines. The goal of holistic practitioners is not only to listen more fully, but in particular to arm patients with tools for more healthful lives. They aim to cure if possible, certainly to delay death, but foremost to view illness not as punishment but partnership.

The key is choice: the freedom to make intelligent and informed decisions about personal health and wellness. Such wisdom comes from recognizing the link between mental and physical health. Triggering the body's natural healing powers is the popular message of leaders in the field of mind/body medicine, including author, physician, and lecturer Deepak Chopra. Through several best-selling books and the lecture circuit, his message has become mainstream: Health means enhancing quality of life. Well-being is not the mere absence of disease, he says, but the dynamic integration of environment, mind, body, and spirit.

Dr. Christiane Northrup, author of *Women's Bodies, Women's Wisdom*, says healing comes from honoring our bodies. She advocates the need to acknowledge the unity of mind and body as well as the powerful role of the human spirit in creating health. Avoiding disease is not the pathway to health, she says; it comes by respecting and caring for oneself, by developing the skills and behaviors associated with true health.

Other leading mind/body proponents, such as Drs. Andrew Weil and Dean Ornish, also focus on the natural rather than the synthetic. According to Dr. Weil, the body has a healing system that works at every level of being; Western medicine's myopia is focusing on disease, on form and structure, rather than on the body's natural gifts. Dr. Ornish puts similar theories into practice in a low-tech program of low-fat vegetarianism, meditation, group support, and yoga. It has shown enough positive results that it is now covered by many major insurance companies as an alternative to heart surgery. Emotional support is also critical: Dr. Ornish believes that when people express their feelings, their health thrives.

Treatment avenues include:

~ Massage therapy and deep tissue body work
~ Acupuncture and Chinese medicine
~ Vitamins and herbs
~ Vegetarianism
~ Aromatherapy
~ Yoga and meditation

~   Stress reduction, biofeedback, and visualization

According to Dr. Kenneth Pelletier, author of books on alternative medicine, older people are more likely to use such methods because they have more chronic conditions, which are not well managed by the current biomedical model of health care. And so this group supplements conventional medicine, where patients are passive recipients, with corollary practices where they take responsibility for their health—to boost the immune system, to relieve stress and chronic pain, and to reduce blood pressure.

Critical to this integrative approach is the difference between *healing* and *curing*. Cure eliminates evidence of the disease and does not necessarily change a lifestyle. Healing, on the other hand, is an inner process by which a person returns to wholeness. This can take place at any level, eliciting greater communion with life.

The Wellness Centers, a nationwide chain, are guided by the philosophy that patients who actively participate with health care professionals in their cancer treatment may promote recovery but certainly will improve the quality of their lives. All services are free. Strategies include stress control, directed visualization, humor, nutrition, exercise, seeking family harmony, and dealing with anger and self-blame. Here psychotherapy is an adjunct to conventional medicine; the mind/body connection is the cornerstone of the program, which emphasizes both psychological and social support. "You are not helpless in your fight for recovery," says founder Harold Benjamin. With participation and support, with changes in unhealthful ways of reacting to stress, the strength to fight is restored.

Michael Lerner, a pioneer in alternative medicine and president of Commonweal research institute in Bolinas, California, says curing is what doctors do to get rid of disease; healing is what patients do in a deeply personal process of safeguarding the soul. The role that each of us can play in our own healing extends beyond therapy to choices about how we live each day. Therefore, he suggests, the more options we have to deal with distress and crisis—including hope— the greater our psychological health will be. Energy—and health— follow thought.

Energy Medicine

One holistic practice is "energy medicine." This discipline suggests that human beings are energetic vibrational fields beyond the five senses. The immune system, for example, is seen as a much larger network connected directly to this energy field and affected by emotions that significantly enhance or suppress its functioning—leading to health or illness. Thus each person bears responsibility for health and balance by how he or she deploys energy in relation to events.

In her work as a medical intuitive, author and lecturer Caroline Myss has observed how and where humans focus their energy and, consequently, how they are either drained of it or supported by it. When you invest in the maintenance of negative thoughts and memories, including grief and regret, depression, anger, guilt, and anxiety, she says, "you are financing the dead of your life with the life of your life." Where fear is in control, the energy of life no longer nurtures. The body then draws on cell tissue for maintenance, resulting in stress, illness, and compromised immune systems.

Health arises out of a process of self-examination, Dr. Myss says, a psychology of pathology. The external world—tribal culture, family, group—determines our beliefs and attitudes until we regain our will power to make choices out of love, compassion, and charity. In examining our rote behaviors and attitudes, we discover how we drain energy by seeking confirmation and attention or by building up our self-image, activities that are dictated by trying to conform to an outside standard. Instead, she says, well-being comes from rechanneling our energy into expressing who we really are. True personal power and the ability to overcome poor health and addiction are within reach: intuition is the guide, available once we are willing to look honestly at ourselves and live more mindfully.

Meditation

Quieting the mind to a stillness that reflects our essential nature is the goal of meditation. It is the basis for a world-renowned program at the Stress Reduction Clinic in Worcester, Massachusetts. Jon Kabat-

Zinn, director of the clinic, is a pioneer of these classes for people with cancer and other life-threatening diseases. Over an intensive eight weeks, participants learn mindfulness meditation and apply insights to chronic stress, pain, and illness. "Mindfulness is vast, because it is fundamentally about wakefulness, about paying attention in one's life—all of it," he writes in *Handbook for the Soul*. "It is simply a universal vehicle with which to explore deep inner connectedness—to access one's own resources for growing, healing, and self-compassion. We use meditation to help nourish the whole of us, both human and divine."

As Sogyal Rinpoche says, "Meditation is bringing the mind home, releasing any tension or struggle, and relaxing into the clarity and peace of your true nature." This focused awareness illuminates the turbulence and suffering created by our thoughts, which parade before us in a numbing stream of inner monologue. Meditation teaches observation of these patterns rather than judgment or reaction to them; it is a method of calming both mind and heart so that compassion, rather than fear, can reign.

It takes practice; mastery does not happen all at once. We must learn empathy for ourselves first, exposing tiers of encrusted habits. Caregiving is an opportunity to look at these layers, meditation practice a tool to do it safely. It is a support system that needs nothing but the willingness to find our own counsel and then trust that it will lead where we need to go.

The key to fruitful meditation practice, says Stephen Levine, is kindness. "Has the practice made the person kinder, more available to speak from the heart? Meditation allows us to cultivate the ability to respond and break the compulsion to react. Meditation in its very essence is the cultivation of responsibility."

If we dwell only in our own world, we remain blind to the universe. For we can never find the way out of suffering if we insist on keeping it to ourselves. It is not that we have deliberately cut ourselves off from the heart of connection; but we have done so carelessly. And now we are asked, in the task of caring for our loved one, to find that place within that touches and heals, that risks and gives. We are asked to leave our islands and come home, where others are waiting for us. We are asked to become part of something larger than ourselves. And everywhere are bridges over which we can make that happen.

CHAPTER 11

Caregivers, Religion, and Spirituality

Well, let us on! We'll plumb your deepest ground,
For in your Nothing may the All be found.—Goethe, *Faust*:
Part II, Act I

It has been told that it was awareness of—and meditation on—old
age, sickness, and death that brought the Gautama Buddha to enlightenment. In societies that view elders as noncontributors to
the marketplace, the wisdom of age cannot teach us how to care for
each other. In a youth-obsessed world, older age gives perspective to
fragmented lives and holds the best hope for connecting with what
endures. Contemplating illness and death opens the passageway to
compassion. In this light, aging is not considered a process of wither-
ing and decline but of ripening and maturation: a life bearing fruit.

This chapter looks at teachings on grief and loss from major wisdom traditions, beginning with Judaism because that is my background.
Although their words differ, their vision remains single: compassion,
integrity, generosity of spirit, and selfless service are the foundation
for inner peace. In my own search for meaning in caregiving, I often
returned to these teachings to find new truths on each turn of the spiral.
They brought welcome perspective to this unwieldy rite of passage

and continue to give solace and direction in the most unexpected ways. These teachings prosper in the presence of human suffering and ensure that the nature of caregiving reflects the highest values of humankind.

Judaism

Lord, what is man, that thou regardest him? or the son of man, that thou takest account of him?
Man is like to vanity; his days are as a shadow that passeth away.
—Psalm 144: 3, 4

In the morning he flourisheth, and sprouteth afresh; in the evening he is cut down, and withereth.
So teach us to number our days that we may get us a heart of wisdom.—Psalm 90: 6, 12

In the throes of grief, Jews are admonished to be mindful of the preciousness of life. Death is very much alive in mourning rituals, which are honed into an artful practice for every stage of bereavement. The body is buried within three days, in plain cloth and coffin, as befits a humble servant. Mourners in the immediate family rend a garment to mark the tear in the fabric of life that this death has wrought. They then sit *shivah* in the home; they neither leave nor work. For the first week, a *minyan* (ten adults) comes to the house for morning and evening prayers; visitors pay respect to the deceased and honor the family, bringing food as a *mitzvah*, or good deed. The significance of the seven days is clear: the world was made in a week and each person is a world, a world that never was before and never will be again.

The cornerstone of Jewish mourning is the *kaddish*, the prayer for the deceased. Devoid of pity—it makes no reference to death—it is instead a glorification of the Lord, a supplication for peace upon the House of Israel. This benediction exhorts Jews to submit to divine will: "When the dark grave swallows what was dearest to us on earth, it is then that Judaism bids us say: 'It was God Who gave this joy unto us; it is God Who hath taken it from us to Himself. We will not wail, nor murmur, nor complain. We will exclaim, 'Blessed be the Name of the Lord.' "

Filial piety is entwined in these verses; saying kaddish is a reverential act even among the nondevout. Formal mourning may continue another thirty days or for a year, if the deceased is a parent. Children recite the prayer three times a day for the next eleven months, limiting social activities as well, and then once a year on the *yahrzeit*, or anniversary of death. Judaism forbids mourning beyond one year: the Talmud, or book of wisdom, instructs Jews not to indulge in sadness, because life is sacred.

The kaddish goes beyond immediate grief to address a key problem surrounding suffering itself: loss of faith. We wonder how a God could be just when loved ones are allowed to suffer and die. This prayer responds in its poetry: God's creations are magnificent and holy; there is an inherent pattern and plan beyond human will; and it is a Jew's obligation to foster peace on Earth in his or her lifetime.

Mourning rites are a framework not just of comfort but also of philosophy; prayers address eternal questions of how to find strength and meaning in times of loss. These pathways are communal as well as personal: friendship and family are vital in the healing process, reminding us that we are not alone in our sorrows. Rites admonish the bereaved to become aware of being part of something greater than grief. A companion memorial prayer asks that the soul of the deceased, which has gone to repose in the wings of the Shechinah, or presence of God, be bound up in eternal life. Thus it is the mourners, facing the reality of death, who proclaim the ultimate meaning of human existence.

Since ancient times there has been a holy society, the *hevra kadisha*, whose function is to prepare the dead for burial. It is a sacred honor to wash the body and say prayers, the last good deed one human can do for another. Today there are new institutions that also take care of survivors, in the form of Jewish hospice and healing centers. Based in teachings that guide practitioners in understanding the benefits of prayer, visits, and religious faith, the Jewish healing movement provides spiritual care to the ill, to caregivers, and to mourners through service, education, training, information, and referral. Rabbis—both male and female—schooled in pastoral care make house calls, visit long-term-care facilities, and comfort families of the terminally ill. There are also support groups for Jewish physicians and mourners, bereavement camps, and training for volunteers who wish to visit the sick.

According to the Talmud, the Shechinah dwells over the head of those who are ill; visiting them is a commandment from the daily prayer service. It is considered a tremendous spiritual boost for the one who performs it. Caring for the sick connects with the sacred heart that binds the family of man and helps establish the Kingdom of Heaven on Earth. It is a joyful obligation that merges with the ultimate task of one who chooses this path: to be *amsagolah*, a light unto nations.

In the film *Schindler's List*, the Holocaust's surviving Jews and their families pay respects at Oskar Schindler's grave site, where they place stones, rather than flowers, on the marker. This custom is a significant symbol of faith in the goodness of the human heart amid the most barbaric tortures. Stones confer solidity, reminding us that memory is, indeed, everlasting. There is permanence in the pain; "while other things fade, stones and souls endure."

Christianity

> If you bring forth what is within you, what you bring forth will save you. If you do not bring forth what is within you, what you do not bring forth will destroy you.—Attributed to St. Thomas

Jews believe that the world is upheld by three pillars: the Torah or book of law, divine service, and deeds of lovingkindness. These are also the foundation of Christianity, focused in the mandate to "love thy neighbor as thyself." Devotional service is the highest expression of these ideals, magnetizing heaven to earth. To fulfill that order, however, we first must love, and forgive, ourselves. This healing transformation is the promise of resurrection—the coming back to life—through giving of one's total being.

Forgiveness comes on the heels of understanding. Jesus told his followers to not dwell in grief, for only the flesh has gone away: "Go bury your deep woes, and smile at grief, and lose yourself in helping others dry their tears." There is one eternal force and that is divine love, the power of the Kingdom of Heaven within. But to make that energy come alive, it must be fed each moment; it must be given sanctuary. Man is the master of the soul, Jesus said; when he has risen up from doubt and fear, he can cleanse his house and bring the tenant back again. Service activates this Christ energy in the heart, for it is not sacrifice to idols that liberates, but the mystery of universal love: "If you would serve the God who speaks within the heart, just serve your near of kin, and those that are no kin, the stranger at your gates, the foe who seeks to do you harm."

Christianity's commandments are clear: truthfulness, forgiveness, acceptance, kindness, selflessness. Herein lies salvation: to make one's ego-centered personality so small, so childlike, so free of all it has collected while journeying through life that it can slip through the eye of a needle into Paradise. It is the rebirth of man as spirit on earth, empty of all but awe and gratitude for every living moment. In this abundance we are free to give; giving becomes, in fact, an irresistible imperative. It is our true nature.

Many congregations are addressing spirituality and aging through national organizations that bring hope and friendship in trying times. Through Shepherd's Centers, elders provide volunteer services to other elders, including home repair, home-delivered meals, and transportation. The National Federation of Interfaith Volunteer Caregivers links community churches to provide social services to frail elders and disabled people in their homes. Senior Adult Ministries support elder congregation members in a full range of religious and social activities that honor older life and wisdom. The Ministry to Nursing Homes trains volunteers from many congregations to provide church services in convalescent facilities and to arrange one-on-one visits with residents. The Presbyterian Older Adult Ministry Network fosters programs to support elders who need compassionate listening.

Christianity's moral code ultimately promises triumph over loss and grief. When we are stripped of things carnal, when we cease to trouble about material goods, what endures is love. Whoever would be great must minister to all: "The highest seat in heaven is at the feet of him who is the lowest man of earth." This is the wealth of manifested life, and of eternal life. This is true freedom, for there are no chains that can bind the creative force of the universe.

Buddhism and Hinduism

> No suffering, however dreadful, is or can be meaningless if it is dedicated to the alleviation of the suffering of others.—Sogyal Rinpoche, *The Tibetan Book of Living and Dying*

Buddhist thought on the nature of suffering and loss is based on the Four Noble Truths, said to be the first sermon preached by the enlightened Buddha. This doctrine states that life is suffering; that desire creates suffering through both clinging and aversion; that suffering can be transcended; and the way is the Noble Eightfold Path. This is the Middle Way between perception of opposites such as good and evil or love and fear, and leads to clear vision, wisdom, insight, and bliss, or Nirvana. The goal is not only a release of suffering but also union with supreme spirit.

Buddhism has an especially close relationship with death as one of the interlinking realities: life, death, after-death, and birth. A soul journeys through these states, or *bardos*, guided by ritual and teachings on the nature of mind and of the awakened mind that lives beyond death. Aspirants are instructed in an inner science leading to enlightenment. In *The Tibetan Book of Living and Dying*, Sogyal Rinpoche says the bardo teachings show precisely what will happen if we do not prepare for mortality: "If we refuse to accept death now, while we are still alive . . . we will remain imprisoned in the very aspect of ourselves that has to die. This ignorance will . . . trap us endlessly in . . . that ocean of suffering."

Today these teachings have been brought to the doorstep of the sick and the dying through means such as Zen hospice and the Rigpa Fellowship. The latter is a Tibetan Buddhist organization that sponsors Spiritual Care for Living and Dying. Here practices are taught for dying and for after-death states, techniques not just for practitioners of Buddhist psychology, but for anyone wishing to explore the enigma of death. Especially there is an emphasis on forgiveness, to purify ourselves of the attachment to our deeds and prepare for the journey through death.

Author Christine Longaker, who teaches these courses in spiritual care, writes in *Facing Death and Finding Hope:*

> The path of life is already a journey toward death, and once you decide to make that journey a spiritual one, then every aspect of your life, including your caregiving work, gives a positive momentum to your spiritual path. Reflecting in your daily meditation on the suffering of all beings, and praying deeply that you might be able to relieve their suffering, is one way of training the mind in compassion. . . . Your [caregiving] work is a very potent form of spiritual practice.

Caregiving is both a devotional path and an active path of service. It embodies a code of conduct prescribed by the great Hindu text, the *Bhagavad Gita.* In this story, the hero, Prince Arjuna, is sickened by what he must do on the battlefield and refuses to go on to slaughter his enemies. Lord Krishna appears and instructs that only the physical form, not the indwelling Self, meets an end. Arjuna is given a divine eye that reveals the essential nature of the cosmos—life's impermanence—and is transformed by the vision of eternal unity.

"Even as a person casts off worn-out clothes and puts on others that are new," he is told, "so the embodied Self casts off worn-out bodies and enters into others that are new. . . . Eternal, all-pervading, unchanging, immovable, the Self is the same forever." By fixating on the outcome of his deeds, Arjuna remains trapped in illusion; in surrendering all action to a higher power, with an intent devoid of selfishness or personal gain, love, or hatred, he is aligned with cosmic truth and freed from suffering. In the sacrifice of attachment to results, he arrives at knowledge of the truth of existence, a union of divine and human aspects. It is a mystic experience: to be in the world but not of it, yet to regard the pain and the joy of others as one's own.

Islam and Sufism

Good deeds, kindnesses, forgivenesses, tolerance, acts of love—
none of these are ever lost, and some day will return to us.—Hazrat
Inayat Khan, *In an Eastern Rose Garden*

Islam was founded on the creed that a higher unseen power controls
an individual's destiny. The reason for existence, the meaning of
life, is serving the will of the one God, Allah. Beliefs and ways of life
are ordained through the Word of God, the *Koran*, revealed to the
Prophet Muhammad almost fourteen hundred years ago. The tenets
of Muslim faith, such as accountability on the Day of Judgment, infuse daily life. The key to Paradise is piety: remembering God through
continual prayer softens the bitterness of death and builds an eternal
bridge over the fires of hell. Solidarity is also fundamental: the spiritual mantle of Muhammad fell not upon a church but on the whole
community.

A mystical branch, Sufism, teaches that God is loving, succoring;
through piety and asceticism, then through joy and love, the pilgrim
transcends the self. In Sufism, the spiritual life is a self-directed journey, following God's commandments, that leads to consciousness of
harmony with spirit—the path is the way to the heart. Through stages
of repentance, abstinence, trust in God, and satisfaction, the Sufi is
raised to a higher plane of consciousness. The work is to transmute
desire into heart, heart into soul, and unify the three into one. It is the
sincere intent of one's acts that matter; their importance lies in the
heart.

Mysticism and Shamanism

Then I sought solitude, and here I soon became very melancholy.
I would sometimes fall to weeping, and feel unhappy without
knowing why. Then, for no reason, all would suddenly be changed
and I felt a great, inexplicable joy, a joy so powerful that I could

not restrain it . . . I became a shaman, not knowing myself how it came about. But I was a shaman. I could see and hear in a totally different way.—An Eskimo shaman

Mysticism is loosely defined as that which is beyond human comprehension; a path of awareness is mystical if we gain access to our hearts. Author Sophy Burnham says there is no way to go on an inner journey without surrender of the selfish ego; yet in the darkness of yearning for fullness, one can find joy. A mystical experience can be a subtle or dramatic meeting with divinity, she says, but the important questions to ask are: Did it make you more aware in the world? Did it make you more compassionate?

Shamanism is a traditional spiritual path in cultures worldwide. Like Buddhism, it is an effort to understand mankind's place in the universe and "the mystery of participation," writes deep ecologist Joan Halifax in *The Fruitful Darkness*. These seers and healers—women as well as men—have gone to superhuman ends, entering altered states of consciousness at will through physical, emotional, and psychological ordeals prescribed by millennia of initiatory practice.

Shamans are messengers between realities, bringing back the wisdom and power to help and heal. Their trajectory is a descent into suffering in order to be transformed. Shamans know the terrain of this Lowerworld; they have journeyed through disease and illness. Because they learn the art of dying, they also know the art of healing and are called "wounded healers." Once weak, the shaman is now strong; once blind, now he sees. He is consummately capable of leading the sick through this land—even through death—guided by a connection with the cosmos. Intuition and compassion are the governing forces in this quest for self-empowerment, but the intent of leadership is to help others rather than to benefit the self.

Shamans—also known as "medicine men" or "witch doctors" to Western minds—are guardians of a body of ancient techniques used to achieve and maintain maximum well-being and an impeccable life. Methods that include shamanic journeying, the vision quest, song and trance dance, ritual objects, and magical words are similar in cultures the world over—in North and South Americas, Africa, Siberia, and Australia—and have been so for thousands of years. Their uniformity indicates the availability of a common path to personal mastery, an ability to develop the inner mind for physical health and healing. Author and practitioner Michael Harner writes in *The Way of the Shaman*:

> Shamanism is a great mental and emotional adventure, one in which the patient as well as the shaman-healer are involved. Through his heroic journey and efforts, the shaman helps his patients transcend their normal, ordinary definition of reality, including the definition of themselves as ill. The shaman shows his patients that they are not emotionally and spiritually alone in their struggles against illness and death. . . . The shaman's self-sacrifice calls forth a commensurate emotional commitment from his patients, a sense of obligation to struggle alongside the shaman to save one's self. Caring and curing go hand in hand.

Family therapist Alexandra Kennedy works with several shamanic techniques to handle grief as a process of liberation. "To the imagination, death is not an ending, not a catastrophe, but a transformation. Within you, your loved one lives on and, with your participation, your mutual relationship will grow and change," she says. Regret, guilt, unfinished business can all be dealt with in the privacy of one's inner world through dreaming, letter writing, dialogues, and imagery. It is never too late to reconcile; the connection is always available.

Wounded healers take many forms today, from those who have had near-death experiences to everyday heroes who return from secret terrors with greater empathy for others. They are the ones with a willingness to share knowledge of the way out of despair, even just one step, for they have peered into the mystery, survived, and found the experience life-changing.

"If we were able to understand sickness and suffering as processes of physical and psychic transformation, as do Asian peoples and tribal cultures," writes ethnopsychologist Holger Kalweit in *Dreamtime & Inner Space*, "we would gain a deeper and less biased view of psychosomatic and psychospiritual process and begin to realize the many opportunities presented by suffering and the death of the ego."

Spirituality and Aging

Whether because of millennium madness or midlife mindfulness, a renaissance of spiritual seeking is bringing ideals into more practical focus. Synchronistically, the arena of family caregiving has become a proving ground as spirituality and aging dovetail into a new quest for meaning and serenity. It is a time to probe what it means to grow older, to reorient life's purpose in the birthplace of death. Gerontologists are finding a link between religious commitment and good health among older people, making it an element in new views about successful aging.

Marita Grudzen, head of Stanford University's Division of Family and Community Medicine, says that caregiving is so demanding, a spiritual connection is critical to the heart of the work. "Especially today in health care, people are doing more with less, and we're confronted with our limitations as never before. Many of us realize that when we come from a spiritual center, we find more peace and satisfaction in what we're doing, and we accomplish things more easily. Spirituality certainly is a counterpoint to burnout."

The quest is to realign with the soul. Religion prescribes the rites of conduct, the rituals and moral values that lead to transcendence. Spirituality addresses transformation itself, riding the flow of time and giving grace to human endeavors. Spirituality and aging are concurrent paths for those who choose to turn to the inner life in search of a better life. In prayer and meditation, in ritual and in deep listening, we find a new rhythm. We detach from what is no longer relevant and prepare for a more universal dream.

Reflecting about death is particularly instructive for those coping with aging and end-of-life issues. Rabbi Zalman Schachter-Shalomi observes, "It is really difficult to spend your elder years if you don't have 'elder mind.' You can't run your elder years with the software of your youth." Later on the pace is slower, the tasks are different: to harvest life, to mentor the next generation, to preserve the wisdom so it doesn't get lost. This is the essence of both religion and spirituality: to sanctify the *full* range of human endeavors.

A Hasidic saying teaches that before we can be together, we must learn to grieve together. Emptied of delusions, we find the purest meaning of relationship, beyond blood ties and social obligation. No matter what a person's religious beliefs, at life's core is spirituality: the connectedness that each of us feels when we understand the true power of relationship.

The lessons of family caregiving confer a joyful way of living that ripples out into the world in deeds both large and small. The message of all spiritual leaders throughout history has been that the individual must learn to transcend selfish concerns to align with a larger purpose. Then we can add to the kindness and the wisdom of the world, that we may all be free of suffering.

CHAPTER 12

End-of-Life Concerns

A dying man is considered the same as a living man in every
respect.—Jewish law

I n Native American tradition, a warrior would choose a good day
and place to die. In modern Western culture, we choose neither
the day nor, often, the surroundings. When we come to the end,
technology straps us to tubes and ventilators in defiance of mortality.
Setting us up for the unkindest cut of all, the medical establishment
pronounces that death is an outrage, that life must be prolonged at
any cost.

The end of life is now center stage for a new ethical agenda. The
nature of the physician-assisted suicide debate, mercy or legalized
murder, is beyond the scope and intent of this book. But its impact and the real-life scenarios that play out around it—especially
the fear of dying in pain—affect families every day. These experiences
can be bitter, yet they can also lead caregivers to conclude that life
cannot be solved, only experienced and cherished. As French
palliative care psychologist Marie de Hennezel writes in *Intimate
Death*, end-of-life work is about "the spiritual labor that goes on inside every dying person: an effort to give birth to oneself completely
before leaving."

Ethical Issues

Personal care of the dying left the homestead about fifty years ago as advances in medical and nursing science brought the possibility of delaying death, or even preventing it, if a person received adequate care in a hospital. By the 1980s, most dying occurred outside the home. Yet in recent years this trend has been reversing because of advances in home-based technology, the desire of families to care for their loved ones at home, the growth of the hospice movement, and greater attention to end-of-life issues. But, according to the Alliance for Aging Research, the majority of older women in North America still die in nursing homes or hospitals.

Death is coming out of the closet as moral concerns surface over both pro-life issues and assisted dying. They provide a forum for examining our values because they force us back on assumptions about what matters when everything is about to be taken away. These are more than legal issues: at their core they are profoundly spiritual, because they raise questions about the purpose of life and the message of death—and what a "good death" truly means.

Today a new conscience awareness is being forged out of urgency. The dialogue on dying is not limited to terminal care but extends to the sacredness of life itself. Humankind has never before been at this crossroads. People are living so much longer—technology is so advanced—that decisions about prolonging life are having to be made among family members who always expected such matters to be the sole domain of medicine or religion.

Rather than feeling buoyed by the medical system, however, they are faced with extremes of decision making: treat the loved one or let him die. "The system makes it scary to make choices because the alternative sounds like abandonment," says Dr. William Knaus, who worked twenty years in the intensive care unit at George Washington University Medical Center in Washington, D.C. "Why do physician-assisted suicides even exist? Because people are afraid of the system, afraid that it doesn't know when to stop. They're afraid of how they're going to die."

Today, dignified care means taking responsibility. There are many subjective areas about which decisions must be made: quality of life, capacity versus incapacity, hospitalization versus treatment at home or in assisted care, hydration or intravenous fluids, psychiatric care or psychotropic medicine. Monitoring care means listening to the whole family, not just reading a medical chart. It is no longer a matter of what can be measured, but of what is most merciful.

Physician and gerontologist Christine Cassel calls modern-day practice "stranger medicine"—where a doctor doesn't know the patient, yet is asking family members if they want their mother to be kept alive. She says, "I think it's unrealistic to ask a family to make that kind of decision and to feel that somehow it was their burden that this happened. The mother's going to die; it's just a question of when. But it's posed as a choice that somehow the family has to make."

Across all ethnic, religious, and cultural lines, North Americans are more afraid of how they may die in today's health care system than they are of death itself. In a recent study, respondents said that the current system does not support their ideal concept of dying. They worry about being hooked up to machines, especially in a nursing home. They fear becoming a burden to their families, yet they would rather not discuss dying because the subject is so unpleasant. They don't feel close to doctors—in fact do not trust them, especially if they have to see a different one every time. They wish to be pain free and to die at home unencumbered by machines and surrounded by loved ones. At least, that is the ideal.

Several studies have found that inadequate training in the health industry, a lack of advance care planning, and uninformed attitudes about dying were resulting in needless suffering. The SUPPORT report said that almost half of seriously ill patients were in severe pain in their last days and that efforts to prolong lives too often merely prolonged dying. This left many of them alone, neglected by their doctors and attached to machines. Dr. Joanne Lynn, a study co-author and director of the Center to Improve the Care of the Dying at the George Washington University Medical Center, says:

This study confirms widely held public fears that death is often difficult and undignified. American culture has a profoundly dysfunctional way of thinking about dying. We live so long while dying now, and it can be such a valuable time. It is clear that we could do much, much better at alleviating pain, reducing isolation, and following the patient's wishes at the end of life. . . . This may require a significant change for all of us in how we think, teach, and talk about end-of-life issues.

For more than two thousand years, the practice of medicine has rested on the Hippocratic oath: to prolong life and to relieve suffering. Sometimes, particularly at the end of life, these two vows seem diametrically opposed. Western medical culture sees death as failure, a view that complicates caregiving in an effort to "do no harm." A society in denial cannot recognize the family problems that accompany death and dying, such as pain and suffering and financial burdens. Caregiver advocates are at the forefront of new ethical quandaries:

~ Which should take priority, prolonging life or relieving suffering?
~ When does existence take precedence over quality of life?
~ Should we employ extreme measures to keep our loved ones alive?
~ Do we have the "right" to die?
~ How will a reform-driven health care system affect dying?
~ Will someone other than family—like the insurance industry—be making these decisions for us?

Current medical technologies allow far more people to survive for long periods and with more debilitating physical and mental capacities, including a vegetative state. These conditions pose dilemmas for those responsible for care. Families as well as health professionals must decide what constitutes appropriate medical care and whether such treatments provide any benefits, or whether prolonged intrusive procedures become burdensome—including intravenous fluids and stomach tubes.

Dr. Timothy E. Quill, an author and primary-care internist in Rochester, New York, who has been prominent in the physician-assisted suicide debate, says, "this whole notion that medical technology has extended life wonderfully . . . has also extended death in ways that aren't so great. As a result, people see others die in ways they don't want for themselves. This leaves them with two fears regarding their own end of life: What if I can't express what I would want? What if I say what I want, and people won't listen because I'm not saying what they want to hear?"

Vicki, forty-one, a mother of two preteens and a former long-distance caregiver, was torn apart by the choices she was required to make.

> The absolute hardest thing was to be the one who decided to let my mom go, and then sit by her side while she died. Because my dad was no longer in any condition to make decisions during the last six months of Mom's life—he also has Alzheimer's—the nursing home staff asked me to take over her care. Since I had power of attorney for both parents, this wasn't a problem. Still, making life-or-death decisions about any loved one, particularly my mother, was incredibly difficult.
>
> I was the one who made the decision not to put her on a feeding tube. I was the one who made the decision not to send her to the hospital when she got a bronchial infection. I was the one who took the power of attorney and the living will for her to sign when she was first diagnosed, and I was the one who wrote the advance directives for the nursing home at the end of her days. Life as a grown-up is harder than I thought it would be. There are many things a caregiver can do to prepare for the "technical" or "operational" demands. I don't believe any of us is ever totally prepared for the emotional demands.

Underlying ethical concerns are economics: for doctors, hospitals, patients, families, and taxpayers. More Medicare dollars are spent at the end of a person's life than at any other time. With a shift in recent years to a payment system that sets a cap for any particular treatment, the economic incentive is to shift from keeping a person alive in a hospital to allowing the patient to die, or removing him or her to a home setting. With pressure mounting to reduce medical bills paid with public funds, life support for the terminally ill is being questioned; as a result, there are concerns that life-sustaining treatment will be withheld from some patients who want it. It is a debate certain to gather steam as the age wave expands and elders speak out, as in a SeniorNet on-line poll in which more than half of the respondents said they would consider physician-assisted suicides.

Euthanasia

Fifty-year-old Donna had always depended on her mother to be there for her: during her divorce and while raising her four children, one of whom was institutionalized for a time with mental illness. A licensed professional nurse at a state mental hospital for adult retarded, Donna was only thirty-nine when her mother, seventy-eight, suffered a major stroke during a five-way heart bypass. She lapsed into a coma, with only brain stem function. The state of Illinois did not allow a living will at the time.

> I had to go to an attorney to file papers and fight for custody of my mother, to make decisions for her. This took months, and Mom died in the process. Meanwhile I was escorted out of the hospital because they were afraid I was going to disconnect her life supports. I had intended to. The state would not allow us to turn off the respirator until doctors taught her brain stem to breathe. Then I had to sign papers to withdraw nutrition and medical treatment to allow her to die of starvation and disease. I felt I was betraying her because the state would not allow her to die with dignity, as she requested twelve years earlier, when her husband died. Fighting for what she wanted made me feel this was the last thank you for loving me.

Whose death is it anyway? The issue has gained notoriety since publication of Derek Humphrey's controversial *Final Exit*, a best-selling guide that elucidates the growing concern over a moral right to suicide. One of the most volatile concerns is euthanasia, or the ending of life before nature deems it. A poll of doctors showed that only a few are complying with patient requests for pills or injections—but more than a third would prescribe a lethal dose if it were legal. A tangled

bureaucracy now encircles dying: it's no longer just doctors and patients who make decisions; hospital administrators, in-house attorneys,
and risk managers also have a say. Death has become negotiable, rather
than remaining private.

Psychiatrist M. Scott Peck, in *Denial of the Soul*, suggests the term
euthanasia is ambiguous at best as it is unclear who is performing the
act and how it differs from suicide or refraining from heroic measures.
However, on a spiritual level, he raises the one issue that drives deep
into the heart of caregiving: cutting a life short of its natural demise
may shortchange everyone's spiritual growth.

"No matter how great the pressure, no matter how understand-
able and normal the denial of death is, it is not healthy," Peck writes.
"Denial thus virtually ensures that no meaningful communication can
take place between the dying and those close to him or her. . . . You
cannot learn anything from your dying if you cannot even face the
fact that you are dying."

The ongoing debate over the rights of the dying reveals the fine
line between the intentional termination of life and the provision of
palliative care—withdrawing or withholding life-sustaining treatment.
Nowhere is the distinction resolved. A committee of the House of
Lords in Great Britain recommended against changing the law to
permit voluntary euthanasia; of the twenty thousand patients who have
received hospice care there, which includes home supplies of medications to control symptoms, only five have taken their lives. The Angli-
can Church recently approved certain forms of assisted death, including increased dosage of pain killers. For two decades, both
physician-assisted suicide and euthanasia have been legal in the Netherlands, with mixed reviews. The country has moved in stages from
considering assisted suicide to sanctioning euthanasia for terminally
ill patients, then sanctioning the practice for the chronically ill
and the psychologically distressed. The most alarming concern aris-
ing from Dutch studies is the documentation of cases in which about
a quarter of physicians stated they had "terminated the lives of patients without an explicit request." In Australia, where voluntary euthanasia is prohibited by law, one study showed that large numbers of
doctors "are intentionally ending the lives of patients," and not always
with consent.

In the United States, physician-assisted suicide is illegal in every state but Oregon. Recently the U.S. Supreme Court handed down a decision long awaited by advocates of both the right-to-die and the pro-life movements. It ruled that terminally ill patients do not have a constitutional right to doctor-assisted death. It left the door open, however: "Our holding permits this debate to continue," wrote Chief Justice William Rehnquist. The controversy continues among ethicists, politicians, and philosophers over fears that the aged will be pressured to commit suicide to save society from the burden of costly medical treatment or abandonment to a nursing home as the number of people over eighty-five skyrockets.

Hospice and Palliative Care

"Dying well" is the philosophy behind Dr. Ira Byock's arguments in favor of comfort care over assisted dying; he is a pioneer in the fields of hospice and palliative care. His Missoula (Montana) Demonstration Project is dedicated to transforming the environment of death. Pauperizing the dying is a disgrace, a situation that could be alleviated by making hospice care universally available. Without adequately funded palliative care programs, he predicts, it will become physicians' responsibility to recommend assisted dying to those who lack adequate resources.

Beyond this issue, however, is the idea that equates death with suffering and dignity with behavior rather than soul. Byock proposes that dying well enlightens those who regard it as a means for personal growth, a chance to understand the personal, not just the medical, nature of dying. This view encourages people to understand that how we treat the dying is a direct, often dire, reflection of the fact that we have placed more value on technology than on life, and on life at all costs rather than on acceptance of natural cycles.

One of the strongest death-with-dignity philosophies is hospice, a form of palliative care whose primary purpose is to alleviate distressing physical symptoms and address the psychological and spiritual needs associated with the disease process. The goal is for a more comfortable existence without prolonging dying. These services were established in Great Britain in 1967 by Dr. Cicely Saunders; the movement emigrated to North America the following year. Ten years later British Columbia established the first hospice service in Victoria, followed by palliative care hospitals in Montreal and Winnipeg. Hospice now flourishes in most developed nations including Australia, where it supplanted "care of the dying" in the late 1970s. Everywhere, comfort care allows management of dying at home or in a special care facility with attention to well-being rather than curing.

Although some pioneering programs now accept patients at diagnosis, generally a patient enters a hospice program after a doctor confirms he or she has six months or less to live. As a medical practice, hospice mandates interdisciplinary care that includes nurses, social workers, clergy, physical and occupational therapists, doctors, pharmacists, home health aides, counselors, and volunteers. As a humanitarian rather than just a medical practice, hospice treats the person rather than the disease. It trains the family in comfort care and educates about death. There is emotional as well as spiritual support; no one in the family is expected to make this passage alone. There is also a year-long follow-up bereavement program.

Jackie was having a wonderful day. Her spirits were lifted, she was feeling good enough to go outdoors, and her three girls were with her, enjoying the pre-Christmas spirit. It was a high point for the entire family: Jackie, sixty-five, had been battling ovarian cancer for a year and a half. Until hospice came onto the scene six months earlier, her pain had been out of control despite the best efforts of doctors and a home health agency.

But with the right mix of medications and counsel, the family was able to make decisions that were well informed—and deeply loving. One of them was a gift of sacrifice. When it was clear that the cancer was hopelessly advanced, Jackie and Frank's three daughters all left their jobs and families to come back to their parents' home full time until the end, despite having their own children—and grandchildren on the way.

Doctors had been urging hospice care for some time. The decision meant that instead of using traditional medicine in a hospital to try to cure the disease, the team of doctors and nurses would monitor and manage Jackie's pain level at home. The family was taught medical procedures they could administer themselves and were counseled by a social worker and a chaplain as their emotional needs dictated. Volunteers and aides came in to bathe Jackie, and a nurse, on call twenty-four hours a day, also made weekly visits. Daughter Connie says:

> There's a myth that hospice is this gruesome picture of people who look like old-fashioned morticians waiting around for someone to die. But instead, it really is this huge support group of incredibly knowledgeable people. The more *we* did for my mother, the worse she got. But when hospice came in, they went back to basics and got her pain under control first. The minute they took over and changed the medications she started feeling better, even though she wasn't going to *get* better.
>
> When they got behind the scene, even as it got tougher it got easier because of the help. They were exactly what we needed, holding us up and helping us cope even in the last couple of days, gently telling us when it might be time to say our good-byes. I know what it's like to feel you're standing out there alone—then someone comes along with a light and shows you the end of the dark tunnel. It certainly made a huge difference.

As a moral philosophy, hospice is also propelling a subtle but substantial shift in the medical community to reconsider training that teaches death is the enemy. Oncologist Derek Kerr is one of a growing number of physicians who care exclusively for the dying. They are the medical extensions of family caregivers, partners in exploring the edges of life. He explains:

> It's not just delivering medical care, but it's delivering personal care. Generally in medical training the dying person is avoided; the dying person reminds doctors of the limitations of their tools. But that person is calling you to do something that might be healing or comforting, which is the old medical calling that has been forgotten because of the triumph of technology, which is not relevant to the person beyond rescue. Even when a patient

can no longer be helped by those tools, that person greatly appreciates it when you sit down and give of yourself or indicate an acceptance of them as they are, because serious illness is an identity crisis.

So you are there as a healer and a companion, which is the essence of medicine. When you are talking about healing, you are talking about wounded persons; and when you talk about curing, you are talking about disease. The doctoring part is to care for the wounded person; actually, that's the soul of hospice. But the ultimate work has to do with defining the wound or offering care or at least indicating to the person that you see their wound—the suffering—so they don't feel so vulnerable and so alone. You have to find the living in dying.

Conscious Dying

Such "living" has emerged in another pioneering movement from the 1970s, called "conscious dying." It was made famous by one of its cofounders, Dr. Elisabeth Kübler-Ross, who proposed that it was not death we need fear, but not living fully beforehand: "to release our inner selves from the spiritual death that comes with living behind a façade designed to conform to external definitions of who and what we are."

This challenge was taken up by her colleagues Stephen Levine, Ram Dass, and Dale Borglum and has reverberated throughout the world. This psychology goes beyond dignity at the end of life to address the fact that by rushing from death and loss, we have never truly lived.

"One of the remarkable things about confronting death is the depth at which it gets our attention," writes Stephen Levine in *Who Dies?* "If you could fully experience even a moment of being in its totality, you would discover what you have always been looking for." Focusing on our relation to death, we cease bargaining with it. We begin to question what or who dies and what or who lives on. Through mindful attention to each moment we become aware of being more than our physical bodies. Dropping investments in who we thought we were, we unfold into who we truly are. And although we may lament the endings, something more authentic comes into play.

Conscious dying is a way to look at suffering as an opportunity for transformation. Dale Borglum, director of the Living/Dying Project, which trains volunteers to care for the dying as well as confront their own fears about living, believes that service combined with some contemplative practice is a potent path to liberation. He explains:

> When we're confronted with death, whether of a loved one or the loss of an identity or even seeing death portrayed in media, that is a mirror that confronts the place where we are unconsciously holding on to our sense of separation, where we're pushing death away. We can use our relationship with dying, and particularly caregiving, as a way of uncovering fears and hopes and desires that have previously been below our level of awareness. It's not necessarily a fun or an easy thing, but it's one of the most direct things we can do to heal the place where we're divorced from our true nature.
>
> Working with dying becomes work on yourself. If you're just doing this to be a good person, then you're not going to get the deepest gift from that practice, and you're almost assured of burning out. If I'm just coming there to help you, I'm not addressing where you are inexorably being drawn as a dying person, into this space of mystery and nonduality. I'm not being there with you. On the other hand, if I'm only doing the meditation thing, talking about nonduality and not relating to you as a human being, then I'm not dealing with who you are now.
>
> When you're caring for someone who is dying, what is revealed is the places where you are blocking your own compassion, where you're needing to be in control. "The peace that passeth understanding" does not get a lot of encouragement in our society; death is not something that can be understood. So there's a balance that's necessary for doing this work fully, between the human and the spiritual dimensions.

Just as we must let go in order to take this journey, we also must detach in order to return home. The potential for healing, for reclaiming life, lies in mindful willingness to go beyond identifying with the many levels of pain to find our genuine nature beneath them. Steven Levine says:

> Letting go of suffering is truly the hardest work we will do. We can't wait until our mind is clouded and the body wracked with discomfort to do work that seems so impenetrable. There is nothing more joyous than the mind that has fear in it but is not frightened, to watch doubt and not identify with it. Western culture doesn't recognize dying as a state of grace, nor the power of mercy and compassion. Freedom from suffering is when your happiness is no longer dependent on the content of your mind, but on the capacities of your heart. If you're not letting go of it, you're getting buried by it.
>
> As profoundly scary as it is, there is nothing that will protect us from death; if we don't love now, we've blown it. That makes today very precious. Don't ask for favors; just be thankful for what is, and gratitude starts to fill up the nooks and crannies. Our inheritance is an appreciation of our capacity to keep our heart open. To close it is to be in hell; heaven is to be open to it. The mercy of the dying process is that it teaches us that if we meet older age with love and service, it will be a boon beyond imagination. The opportunity for insight is unparalleled. Love is the only rational act.

The illness of a loved one causes us to remember our own fragility, that life is not forever. That information can either overwhelm us or engage us in each moment. The pain of being with those who are dying should not be squandered on frivolous emotions. There are no big or small decisions, the sorcerer Don Juan tells anthropologist Carlos Castaneda in his apprenticeship for freedom: there are only choices we make in the face of our inevitable death.

Former French president François Mitterrand once visited a palliative care unit where he sat at the bedsides of the dying. He was struck by their serenity and pursued a course of inquiry with Marie de Hennezel, the patients' counselor, to learn the sources of strength that erase anguish and fear. He found that with a caring presence that allowed pain and despair to express themselves, at the moment of utter solitude and breakdown "the dying seize hold of their lives, take possession of them, unlock their truth. They discover the freedom of being true to themselves. It is as if, at the very culmination, everything managed to come free of the jumble of inner pains and illusions that prevent us from belonging to ourselves. . . . Death can cause a human being to become what he or she was called to become; it can be, in the fullest sense of the word, an *accomplishment*."

Conscious living entails coming to terms with mortality, past the scared places and the paradox. Caregiving offers a unique opportunity to shift our relationship to aging and death and to the way we commune with all other sentient beings. We invite death as a counselor, giving it space to teach us lessons of patience and gratitude. Understanding the universality of suffering and fear, we no longer sequester our hearts. And life begins again.

CHAPTER 13

Caregiving as a Rite of Passage

In the middle of this road we call our life
I found myself in a dark wood
with no clear path through.—Dante, *The Divine Comedy*

Through the ages, rites of passage have helped humankind to understand our place in the universe and to make peace with it. Rituals and symbols ease major life transitions, explain loss, and celebrate life's glories. They invest the events of life with substance and mark milestones by which we define ourselves, our communities, our realities. They help us see things as they are; they teach us to see things differently.

Ancient peoples, especially in Egypt, Tibet, and Mesoamerica, sought guidance in instructional texts called "books of the dead." These tomes of wisdom maintained man's spiritual link with nature and provided purpose in relation to the cosmos. Today Western culture honors few markers in the life cycle, especially older age, which it sees as a complex series of disorders rather than a time of enrichment.

A rite of passage marks the culmination of smaller turnings: it is the crossing of a liminal threshold, a rotation of consciousness that causes a shift in perspective. Caregiving is one of these frontiers in its power to release illusion. Conventional wisdom gives way to real insight, a melting down of frozen forms that we were taught as children and that have prevented us from crossing into spiritual maturity. According to philosopher Friedrich Nietzsche, the uplifting of soul comes by fulfilling the task of killing the dragon whose name is "Thou shalt." When the beast is slain, the child is free of the rules and restrictions of society and history; the child has mastered the forces of civilization and may use them to *live* life rather than submit to it.

Myths and Rites of Passage

Myth and mystical tales have charted this labyrinth and the help that is available: Dante and his Virgil, who leads him out of the shadow world; the fairy godmother and the helpful crone in European lore; spirit guides who accompany the living over the River Styx in Hades, whose waters are fed by the memories of all past deeds and are poisonous to the living. Princess Ariadne found her way to freedom by only a strand of linen thread; it was fine yet sturdy enough to lead her through. In the Jewish mystical tradition of the Kabbalah, the companion is known as the Shechinah, the female presence said to reside with God from the beginning of creation and who went into voluntary exile with Adam and Eve as an expression of compassion.

Departure from the world is not an error, but the first step on the path to greater life. In *The Divine Comedy*, Dante loses his patriarchal positions of authority and honor at midlife. He is confused, disoriented, lost in a dangerous wilderness. He descends a difficult razor-edged path through levels of Purgatory, working through doubts and purging fixed desires like pride and envy. He learns to trust the unconscious forces at his side: As "terror turn'd/To comfort on discovery of the truth," the poet becomes less fearful, and Virgil, who appears at a critical moment, leads him toward the height. Eventually Beatrice, an initiatory guide, takes him to Paradise, where he becomes illuminated: he learns that the love of God informs the entire universe, even into the darkest realms of hell.

In esoteric Judaism, the sense of displacement and the passage required to return to wholeness are represented by the Shechinah. In this account of creation from the Book of Proverbs, the guardian angel says, "The Lord created me at the beginning of his work, the first of his acts of old." She accompanies those who have lost their sovereignty, guarding the fountain of wisdom and the hope of restoration. On the day exile is ended she is commanded to exchange the garment of sorrow for the glory of God, a reunion of creator and creation.

"The soul world always awaits the novice and the wanderer," writes Clarissa Pinkola-Estés. Thus it is in navigating the mythological River Styx, passing from one state of being to another. The task is to cross the land of the dead "as a living creature, for that is how consciousness is made." We must neither rest on our laurels nor become paralyzed by fears of what may lie ahead. Passage means movement, and movement requires the unexpected.

When we have reached the point at which we are open to change and self-discovery, it is said, these ancient helpers arrive. They are called forth because of adversity and danger; they are also part of who we are. Mythologist Michael Meade writes in *Men and the Water of Life*, "They appear when a certain depth of desire becomes set in the heart and when there is nowhere else to go. The companions are part of the human heritage; they are ancestral forces that become available at the last hour. . . . They are capacities and powers acquired through conscious suffering and a genuine sense of purpose."

What propels us out of darkness is our own psychic momentum; others may lead us to the threshold, but we alone make the crossing into light. No matter that we may be inept to solve every problem: our hearts have opened enough that we are no longer shipwrecked. In our meetings with the unexpected we have arrived at the welcome truth: it *is* possible to find meaning in suffering. Compassion and a more fluid approach to life lead home. We return the way we came but with a new heart, new eyes, and new ears.

Inner Resources

When we become attuned to our soul's desire, a force is set in motion that gathers unto itself a series of events, conspiring in impossible coincidence to help us go on. Initially, incurring great loss, feeling helpless and worthless, the journeyer suffers greatly, a process known as symbolic death. To move forward, help is needed. In the sanctuary of the heart, where the greatest protection and resilience reside, innate wisdom thrives and is waiting to be remembered. According to psychologist Lorna Catford in *The Path of the Everyday Hero*, these resources represent "the deep well of wisdom that the hero has in reserve [and that are also known as] grace."

For a decade, Bob, fifty-two, has taken care of his ninety-year-old mother, who has Parkinson's disease and osteoporosis. There are no relatives nearby, no close neighbors. A computer programmer and engineer, he was able to balance work and care for eight years until he realized he needed to be with her full time. Approaching his duties as an engineering problem, Bob has managed to defuse depression and occasional bouts of anger by observing that his mother lives in the present and that she is not deliberately making life difficult.

When I say things like, "If you do this, that will happen," I might as well be talking Martian to her. I have restructured some of the situations so that triggers for a power struggle are eliminated. Sometimes it is as simple as moving a piece of furniture out of her reach. Although sometimes I have lost patience to the point where I yell and scream, I no longer deal with crises by fretting about things out of my control. The self-recrimination that follows is terrible. But it is unreasonable to expect that I will always be able to repress everything—that will hasten burnout. So I think about the incident constructively afterward, perhaps by restructuring my own attitude. If it isn't something related to safety, maybe the answer is as simple as, "It's not that important, don't sweat the small stuff." I don't always succeed in doing this, but it works often enough for me to continue to try.

My mother is almost completely unlike the person she was. I am a very different person from who I was ten years ago. I know that today's situation would have completely crushed and destroyed that younger me. I am determined to carry out this responsibility in the best way possible, and under these circumstances that is to do most of it myself. The greatest reward is to have found resources within myself that I did not know were there.

We are either trapped by our beliefs or freed by them. To the extent that we grasp and identify with physical reality alone, we suffer. If we resist impermanence, insisting on rote agendas that have no relation to cycles of life and to the profound and holy emptiness that cannot be possessed, we remain unable to feel fulfilled by what we have been called upon to do. But we are not concrete statues. If we can allow for possibilities, then we will not get caught up short when major change is heralded.

There is incredible potential for freedom in the human heart that leads not away from the world but toward compassion, no matter what happens. What it takes is a rededication of intent and patience. Then we may choose, moment by moment, our reaction in any set of circumstances, even if they seem cavernous. Our wider purpose takes us beyond pain and sadness and releases us from the ways that inhibit who we are becoming.

Turning Points

When we can no longer return to the life we knew, the person we were, the direction we came from is shrouded in black. We could not find our way back if we tried. We are compelled to continue on, an urgency that is the key to survival. As we cross this new burning ground of tests and turns, we come to rest in stillness. The task here is to give the lessons of darkness a language of light. The path is narrow, for once again we must choose between the pairs of opposites. And we must choose wisely: one way leads farther into the maze; the other begins the road to freedom.

In *No Enemies Within*, psychologist Dawna Markova highlights this stage of the journey:

A turning point challenges us to decide to reclaim our shadows and resources, to re-perceive the world and our relationship to it, to re-integrate our fragmented selves, and to re-direct our lives.

. . . These fulcrum moments, the experiences that we don't choose, which we might give anything to avoid, provide us with the precious opportunity to reconnect with our souls, to forge an ongoing relationship with our hearts, minds, and bodies. It is here we have the chance to learn the lesson that no one studies willingly—that it is possible to grow from suffering.

Ann suffered a series of traumatic events that culminated in the sudden death of her husband, Dick, from a massive coronary. He was sixty-three and had never been ill; Ann was several years younger. She had recently brought her parents, ages eighty-three and eighty-eight, to live with them because her mother was no longer able to care for her dependent husband. Suffering from agoraphobia and housebound for more than ten years, Ann was shattered. She was incapable of caring for herself, let alone cooking, cleaning, washing, and tending to her parents' needs. She could not maintain her large home, so she sold it and moved into a condo. Friends found a lovely apartment in senior housing nearby where her parents could remain independent.

When Dick died, Ann had almost recovered from her illness, except for driving. She had to learn to put aside her fear; she had no recourse but to function. Ann says she has handled many difficulties since then, including hives, high blood pressure, depression, panic attacks—and occasional thoughts of suicide. Two of their children, accusing Ann of causing their father's death for having burdened him with her parents' care, didn't speak to her for a year.

Her father has died but Ann visits her mother, Minnie, now ninety-two, almost daily. She has found joy in helping others, volunteering for the Red Cross and visiting the sick and dying at hospitals and nursing homes, an activity she and her husband once shared. Although Ann had always felt like a coward because of the agoraphobia, her long-buried personal courage saw her through, and today she no longer pictures herself as weak.

Life is a classroom. If we learn from the trials we are sent, we grow. If I did not believe that God is with me and I am not alone, I doubt that I could have accomplished what I have. I have overcome personal bonds. I have accepted the loss of my best friend. I have cared for my parents. I have become independent. I have given my heart to this task that God has given me.

Surrender is a female quality, along with nurturing and purifying. But the lesser-known side of the feminine is represented by the more earthy aspects of birth, the life cycle, and death. According to Jungian analyst and author Marion Woodman, whose works focus on balancing masculine and feminine, without surrender to higher values—nature, emotions, the source of life, and intuition—there is no life at all.

> We are realizing the power of love to heal. That's an opening of the feminine at a level that we haven't known, and we have no idea where it will go. . . . In the letting go, you invite in the higher order. You don't lose anything. You find something. . . . If we give that a chance, it will take us to wholeness. Our problem is that we intervene because we think we know better.

There comes a time in the kingdom of the dark when dragons are fought and conquered, even when the hero is dismembered or crucified. We cannot overcome our limitations until we are ready; and we can only be ready when we are willing to expand out of moribund patterns. Beyond these tests the seeds of the future are sown. It is where the labyrinth ceases to cast its own shadows and takes on the light of the wayfarer's intent.

"There is a land of the living and a land of the dead and the bridge is love, the only survivor, the only meaning," wrote Thornton Wilder in *The Bridge of San Luis Rey*. A caring heart can free our souls.

Taking Charge

The challenge that has resounded through the ages, in legend, myth, fairy tale, and ritual, is not to dismiss the dark night and return to the "old self," but to find passage all the way to the end of despair where the promise of a better world awaits. The rite involves tests of mettle, a solitary time that develops strength of will we never imagined.

While Tommye and her husband, Bill, then in their sixties, were vacationing in Norway, an infection in one of his legs spread throughout his body. Badly burned at age eighteen, he had been plagued by infection over the years. In a tiny town the new wound became serious; they had to return the next day to Oslo, a ten-hour trip via two trains, a bus, and a harrowing ship-to-ship transfer on planks above a choppy ocean.

But before they could get Bill to a hospital, his leg burst open. Two days later the tour group left without them. Raised an only child and never having made a decision on her own—Bill had always made them, but now he didn't even recognize her—Tommye was alone in a large city, knowing neither language nor geography. Holed up in a Catholic nunnery, she didn't know how many days had passed when five doctors met her in the hospital to convey that Bill wasn't responding to medication. " 'Sirs, you are wrong,' I said. 'I will be taking my husband home. Your problem is finding out how and when I do that.' "

When Bill was well enough to leave, the social services director asked about the couple's assets. Tommye froze; she had no idea what they owed, what the exchange rate was, or even how much money they had. Reaching the point of no return, she had to take charge. She began to improvise. She learned how to open a banking account and transfer funds overseas. She saw to it that doctors in Oslo worked with the Medicare office in Chicago. The banks in Oslo worked with banks in New York. The hospital coordinated with the airlines, and the airlines arranged for ambulances at each stopover. Tommye learned self-reliance at her point of greatest desperation, developing skills that would serve her ten years later when her mother became ill.

On one of the frequent twelve-hundred-mile drives to care for her mother, Tommye had a breakdown. "Everything came tumbling out, along with tears dredged up from a depth I didn't know existed. I was mad because negative things were happening to those I loved and I was unable to do anything about them. I was most angry because I felt so helpless at times when I felt I should have been the strongest."

Tommye's mother passed away shortly after, followed six months later by Bill. Having determined to be strong and bear it all, Tommye became ill and was hospitalized, suffering from depression, sleeplessness, forgetfulness, and the inability to do simple tasks—all signs of deep grief. She had depended on a three-legged support, all of which had collapsed: her parents, her husband, and her job. Suddenly she didn't belong anywhere or to anyone. And yet, realizing that she had herself to rely on, she pulled back from the edge with determination to find a way to surmount her troubles. The turning point came when she stopped grieving for what was lost and began to focus on what really mattered in caring for her loved ones.

> There is no way you can piece together the old life; it is gone. But everything became acceptable because of our love. The more love there is and the deeper that love, the easier it is to find acceptable solutions and to understand those situations for which there are no solutions.
>
> You have a lot more options than you realize. You have to create a new life. I became a much stronger woman than I had been, making decisions and resolving problems. These experiences taught me great compassion for others and more patience when dealing with people who are hurting. Deep love is unconditional; it conquers all things. Maybe caregiving should be called "heart-giving care."

Rites of passage cannot be predicted or guaranteed; any step can lead us off course, just as any can lead us home. Each juncture of the journey offers choice: whether to shut off from the experience or to receive the offering. True to the form of folklore wisdom, we are made whole by our disenchantments, illuminated by our illusions.

Cultural anthropologist Angeles Arrien has charted the great adventure of the second half of life, a time that fairy tales reveal as the return of magic and wonder. Midlife is a chance to resurrect the dream we were entrusted with at birth, to make the "great crossing" and create our legacy. It is a time for reparations and humility, for mercy and grace. "So often we associate the second half of life with illness and depression and giving up and waiting for death to come," she says. "But the truth is that midlife is a threshold where creativity can burst you wide open, and real intimacy finally comes into your life."

Changing Perspectives

In ancient times, crossroads were places of opportunity as well as the abode of destructive spirits, says writer Marc Ian Barasch. Sometimes major change is announced not by thunder and lightning on Mount Sinai, but by a simple shift in attitude. We can't alter the fact that life contains sorrow, but we can change our perspective. It is this expanded awareness—freeing even a micron of stuckness—that establishes the journey home, bestowing the strength to carry on through inevitable hard times. It is what Carl Jung called *"metanoia,"* or a fundamental change of attitude when one looks the monster straight in the eye, and he vanishes.

For Jean, understanding came not so much through the portal of divorce, the end of her own forty-two-year marriage because of abuse, but through reengagement as caregiver to her mother, Dottie. After much heartache, Jean was just getting back on her feet and enjoying being a grandmother when Dottie, eighty-two, began sounding weaker. She has a lung disease similar to emphysema and cystic fibrosis that kills most sufferers by midlife, as well as sinusitis, poor eyesight, and poor hearing. Dottie reported that she didn't feel well enough to prepare evening meals and was going to bed hungry. Meanwhile Jean's stepfather, Bill, seventy-seven, who suffers from hearing loss and lethargy, was having only a bowl of ice cream at night.

So Jean, an only child, decided to help out. She quit two jobs, put her belongings in storage, left her home of thirty years, and moved a thousand miles south. Surprisingly, when she arrived, she found things in order: home-delivered lunches five days a week, a cleaning lady three times a week, a home services aide to give baths two or three times weekly, and a visiting nurse to check vital signs once or twice a week. When Jean called an attorney to check over their wills, he assured her that everything was in order.

Yet she felt they were not eating right or living right, and she told them so. She took over all the grocery shopping and errands and cooked dinner every night. She bought audiobooks to pull them out of their depression. She wanted control, which produced resentment in both directions. But recently Jean had an epiphany. Praying for guidance, she discovered how she was manufacturing her own stress: she had approached caregiving assuming that she was younger and smarter than her parents; she was hell-bent on improving their diets, their home, and anything else she didn't approve of.

Today, with new resolve, she says:

> If the way they live is not to my liking . . . that is why I got an apartment a few miles away! Just who did I think I was? Now I understand that if our roles were reversed, I would not appreciate my children coming in and trying to change the way I have done things all my life. I just learned very quietly that I was not going to change them, and it was me that was going to have to change. I am now more at ease, and since my parents are feeling better, I do only what they ask me to do. Now they are a lot happier, and so am I. I have not had these feelings of thankfulness, kindness, joy, and freedom since before I was married at nineteen.

Flexibility is one of the gifts on the path of return, which is set in motion in this rite of passage. It comes from being more concerned about *doing* right than about *being* right. Case manager Pat Coleman, who has counseled many families in crisis, has found that usually it is the caregiver, not the care receiver, who must change in order to make the situation workable. She says:

> We are fixated that Mom or Dad should behave a certain way because that's what we know. We want our parent to respond the way that parent has always responded. But it's the caregiver who has to change. We have to say, "My mom is dying, and she's dying in this way, and this is the biggest tragedy of my life." When we can go through this process, then we can begin to change.

Rites of passage recover a sense of wholeness and proportion, a frequent archetypal theme in myths and tales where the magic of happiness is possible through new eyes. Artist and author Gertrud Mueller Nelson, who lectures on myths and fairy tales, explains in *Here All Dwell Free*:

Those unfulfilled yet possible fantasies have their place. Through imagination we cultivate what might become possible; we cultivate such fantasies because they represent a primal urge to a restructuring of our whole society and redemption, so that we can finally achieve Home . . . because the return home was the long route around and into and through what had become stuck, repressed, forgotten, handicapped, unfulfilled.

Crossing the Threshold

Obstacles become openings, time and again. Says Yellow in *Hope for the Flowers*, "How can I believe there's a butterfly inside you or me when all I see is a fuzzy worm?" Pal Stripe says she must give up her identity as a caterpillar. "What *looks* like you will die, but what's *really* you will still live. Life is changed, not taken away."

Catherine, age forty, punctuates her story with gutsy laughter and a clear view of what she and her husband went through over seven unbelievable years, starting when she was thirty-one. John suffered from a rare auto-immune disorder that was eventually named after him. It had variations of about eight ailments, including rheumatological polyarteritis. He also had a stroke and a heart attack while doctors were trying to treat the disease, which affected his nerves and moved into his organs, destroying all his healing capacity.

In the first four years, everyone believed the illness would shut off. When they realized it was permanent, doctors started aggressive maneuvers including chemotherapy, transplant medication, and a lot of steroid-type treatments, which inflicted their own side effects. Yet the couple felt it wasn't just John who was sick: they were in that place together.

From the outset all the stages of grief were there, condensed and powerful. There were parts of the marriage forever lost—the ability to show affection, the ability to make love or to show love in a tangible way. Catherine had to take over all the partnership aspects so that even the partnership disappeared. She was responsible not only for taking care of John, but for his life—what an incredibly difficult burden, she thought.

Catherine says John would ask why she didn't just leave him, but she couldn't live with herself if she did. He hadn't gotten sick on purpose, so it was something they had to handle. John worked very hard at not taking out his anger on her. But their relationship, while still very loving, had changed. Catherine was no longer the traditional wife: she was his sister, his nurse, his mother, and his friend—sometimes even his enemy—but rarely his wife. He was a wonderful person, but not the man she married. When John was forty-five, he passed away. They had been married thirteen years, half of which he was ill.

A grief observed has been cathartic; Catherine has looked realistically at their relationship so that healing could take place. There's one side of grief that prepares a person for loss, she says, but there's also devastation to deal with: what could have been, what might have been. In becoming responsible for John's life, Catherine lost any sense of who she had been. There was no time for herself while he was ill; so when he died, she didn't have anything to do.

Catherine entered counseling to make sure she was dealing with everything she needed to, including guilt about hoping his suffering could end and about feeling she somehow had brought on his death. In the grief process she didn't want to put this darkness back into her life, to one day look back with regret or resentment about "losing" seven years. Coming out of intense loneliness, she has been engaged in rediscovery of parts of herself that had been long buried: "It's like getting to know an old friend. Some things I pull out and don't like to look at. But then, oh wow, I remember *this* part of me. It is really exciting, like coming out of a fog."

Catherine looks back on some of her tasks and has no idea how she accomplished them. Although caregiving took its toll physically, emotionally, mentally, and financially, "the spiritual aspect is there if you look for it. Today a lot of things are the same, but I have a different perspective as to what's important in life. I have a much better respect for the fragility of life, and I've done a lot of soul-searching about the choices I've made. I want to make sure that my priorities are really the ones I'd want to have, rather than ones someone else thinks I ought to have."

In *Healing into Life and Death*, Stephen Levine writes, "The toll for crossing to the other shore of wholeness is the relinquishment of our suffering. This crossing over is what is called healing; it costs each of us identification with 'my pain.' It may even mean that our lives will never be the same."

Returning to Life

The point of return, the darkest hour, has been defined in classic literature and in mythology as the beginning of the journey back to our true self. Although we do not wish for the trials that have taken us so far away, they can also be the vehicle that ferries us home. We discover that the road laid out before us is the one we have always been on, but it is much wider now: our limits have been stretched and our hearts can handle more.

The path is both a going and a returning, shaped like an endless hourglass of successive expansions and narrowings. Throughout it we are recapturing what we thought was lost forever, rebuilding a life we thought could never be. We are reborn out of the wasteland of our disenfranchised selves, reclaiming ourselves out of loss. Our perseverance has led us back. We are ready to reenter society, with a new spirit and a new purpose.

In St. John of the Cross's *Dark Night of the Soul*, the soul walks securely even though in darkness, "With no other light or guide/Than the one that burned in my heart." The path of return is harrowing but intensely happy in faith that the result is union with spirit in love. Uncertainty is critical to the process, for it is in that place of unrestricted possibilities that truths are mysteriously revealed in the clear light of divine love.

It is crucial not to take the darkness out of wisdom, says Michael Meade, for wisdom forms in the half-light where the upperworld and the underworld meet. It is attained by going into the depths, probing the matrix of emotions where suffering strips away false connections to put us in touch with the central source of life, where we are all one. Yet we still must cross into new life individually; "the last deed has to be done by oneself," wrote Joseph Campbell in *The Power of Myth*.

The dragon of being bound to one's ego—beliefs, needs, fears, the places where we are unyielding—is slain by unlocking those little rooms where we have preserved the best of ourselves. When we have come full circle, we become the still point at the center. Dynamic compassion becomes the alpha and the omega of our existence.

Fancy Nightmares

In a dream, Mother and Father are sitting on their deck at twilight, an ashen hue to the dusk, the air diaphanous and peaceful. Dad is smoking a trademark cigar, smiling at me as wisps of aromatic smoke waft slowly into the trees. As he flicks the ashes to the ground, staring with a mischievous but knowing grin, he remarks, "We've had wonderful times."

My parents were well-ensconced in a bright, spacious room with a large picture window and decorated in a Southwestern motif. The staff was attentive though Mother could not have twenty-four-hour monitoring except in Arcadia, the secured dementia unit managed compassionately by their new friend Jennifer. Every morning Mom met me, purse in hand, demanding to go home. It must have taken hours, but she was removing plastic liners from the trash cans and pulling her few things out of the dresser, making little garbage baggage. When I would gently try to take it from her, she conjured unbelievable strength to prevent me from spoiling her plans.

I thought Mother kept asking where the mail was, as she had at the condo, but now it seemed excessive. By the third day the reason for her agitation became clear: she was not asking for mail but for *Mel*—having ridden to the nursing home separately, she could not make the cognitive connection that the man in her room was her best friend of fifty years. She believed Mel to be at home and was desperately trying to get back to him. When I asked who she thought was sleeping in the other bed, she burbled, "Some nice gentleman."

I was knocked out by this unexpected twist. Over the days her behavior became more frenetic, and one of her fits startled Father awake. "What's wrong, Elaine!?" my father asked his wife, full of sweet heartache. Some momentary purity in her diction clarified what she was saying, and realizing she didn't recognize him, he broke down. All those years, all that it had taken to keep them together—and now this.

I have always cherished a picture that now hangs in my hallway. It is how I best remember them, how I want to remember them. It is a greatly enlarged snapshot from a vacation in St. Croix, when they were sea-swept and tanned and their sailboat had broken down and was being towed to shore. They were beaming and they were carefree, a fine reminder of their good times until a nursing home orderly came in and asked Dad who was in that picture, unwittingly revealing how much life had changed in so short a time. After that day he believed he was old and knew there was nothing he could do about death. He no longer felt important to the community and began to disappear into his dreams.

I arranged the best care I could, talking with everyone who came in contact with my parents day or night, so grateful they would have proper medical attention. Yet nothing could assuage my guilt that, though this was the only possible decision, it was the worst thing I could have done. When I could coax no further benefit from my visit, it was time to go. My father squeezed my hand so tight, I thought he would crush it. To my surprise, Mom didn't follow me this time; she stayed at the window—waving, smiling, loving, knowing. Even with all this, I never really believed my parents would die. But *I* wanted to die, because of such a lousy ending for two lovely people. In the parking lot I cried for half an hour, until the tears soaked through to my knees.

Yet I began to feel a new season arriving as my parents' lives faded into fall, a cycle that might be possible to survive. My mother's seventy-first birthday arrived on Halloween. Coincidentally, my father's uncle Jake, who had lived in the Arcadia unit for two years with Parkinson's, passed away that day. Dad had barely remembered to tell us; when I said I was sorry, he said, "Don't be. Jake wanted it." As we were talking about all manner of things he suddenly exclaimed, bemusedly, that he was visualizing what we were saying moments before we said it. He was delighted by an awareness other than his linear rationality, and proclaimed, "These sure are some fancy nightmares." They were indeed.

PART IV

Reclaiming Life

CHAPTER 14

Awakening the Heart

The whole world is a narrow bridge, a very narrow bridge, and the main thing is not to be afraid.—A Hasidic saying attributed to Rabbi Nachman of Bratslav

E very day gives abundant opportunity to decide whether to be a victim or to embrace the world. We all suffer in one way or another, yet the fires of hell can ignite the heart. And once love is sparked, although its constancy may ebb and flow, it can never die. It is an uninvited grace that opens our hearts: compassion lives in the here and now and faces outward.

Grief has become initiator and guide, transformed from a numbing weakness into a fount of spiritual expression. "In daily life we must see that it is not happiness that makes us grateful, but gratefulness that makes us happy," says Brother David Steindl-Rast. Here are stories that reveal the power of unconditional love to widen the path and light the way.

Forgiveness

When Alzheimer's struck Tung's mother, it changed their past as well as their future. First her brother stood guard at their mother's house where she lived alone and was in command. Tung didn't think she could handle the caregiving because she and her mother had never had a good relationship. Soon there were family fights, and the situation became more difficult than either child had anticipated. Still, Tung took over care of a woman who had suffered extreme affliction in China and had willed herself to survive in the Old Country before coming to America.

Yet a laundry list of grievances, long simmering from childhood, was never far from mind. The meltdown began one day when Tung brought over her prized Labrador, trained as a wheelchair companion. Her mother was tossing a ball for him. Tung heard frantic barking and found her mother laughing because she had thrown the ball on the roof and loved that the dog was going crazy.

Tung lost her temper, screaming at her not to wreck his self-confidence as she had done with her kids. She laid it out—how her mother had destroyed her children by putting them down for little things, and for big things; how she called them stupid, and made them understand that she was superior; how it was a loss of power to thank her daughter or appreciate anything she did. And so Tung expected to be demolished. Instead, her mother said, "I know. I'm trying to change."

Her mother asked to have a dog, too, but Tung didn't want to be responsible for more crimes. Her mother again said she was going to change. Tung was stunned and skeptical, but she began looking for a dog. Eventually, Tung moved mother and puppy into her own home; then they all went to a more rural area that had plants her mother could tend. But she continued to decline; after an impossible time because of a stroke and a doctor who refused hospice care, she passed away, dehydrated and in pain.

Having a relationship with her mother at the end of life is something Tung never expected. They had become a family, two people and two dogs. They laughed a lot, more than ever because her mother could be silly and fun. She feels they did have a kind of resolution even though they both were angry a lot. But it was all right.

"I was always real thankful for her dementia because it would have been impossible for the rapprochement without it. Things would have been frozen in a very bad state. With it, it was sort of workable. I badmouthed my mother all my life, and then I got a whole different look. It made me feel if this has happened, then anything can happen."

Twelve years ago, after her father passed away, Linda became the primary caregiver for her eighty-six-year-old mother, Marie, who left her home of seventy years to travel two thousand miles west. Despite a history of poor relations, Linda cared for her needs out of duty, but she never felt a bond. Her mother had a history of mental illness and was abusive to Linda as a child. But when Marie was diagnosed with dementia, Linda, fifty-six, decided to mend whatever tears in their relationship she could and to do it with love so she could devote herself to caring in a compassionate way.

For a time she was an emotional wreck, but Linda found a therapist, talked with others about similar experiences, and kept searching until she found answers. She is at peace for the first time in her relationship with Marie, willing to set aside the baggage of so many years and forgive the past.

> We are all so fragile and so sensitive to the conditions around us . . . what else can we do but make our world so small when we are in pain. But allowing the pain to get big enough, then one can reach out and touch a ray of hope from someone, from a book, another caregiver, a group. Caregiving is a temporary stage in a relationship which will take you to a level of compassion that you have never before experienced. It's not the disease—it's the level of *giving* that changes your life.

A Touch of Heaven

Donna was very much in love with her husband, Bryn, who died at age fifty after a year-long battle with pancreatic cancer that had spread to the liver. Only three years earlier they had built a new home, happy to move back to the town where Bryn was born. Ill herself with fibromyalgia, Donna never let her husband know how difficult it became to care for him, even with nursing and housekeeping help. Their five grown children and three grandchildren all spent time sharing their love with him.

Donna's grief is still present, but it has become imbued with magic. Even though there are dark days—waking up in the morning realizing that it has all ended—she feels his presence everywhere and speaks with him often, sensing when his spirit is near. "I can feel his touch like butterflies all over me. He talks with me and gives me answers that I wouldn't dream up. I thought I was just imagining this at first, but one conversation made me realize that these are not my thoughts, even though they are in my head. I had been talking with Bryn and he said he had to go, he had work to do. I laughed and asked what work he could possibly have. He replied, 'I have God's work now.' "

Another time, when Donna was upset and told Bryn how much she missed him and how bad she felt that he was going to miss so much of their kids' and grandkids' lives, he said he was with each of them. That was not a big surprise, but she had become quite upset, crying and sobbing. "He told me to lie still. It felt like my whole body was flooded with—I don't know how to describe this feeling; I was so amazed. I asked him what he had done. He replied, 'I just gave you a little bit of heaven.' "

Finding Equanimity

Film editor Deborah Hoffmann wrestled at length with an inability to accept the changes that dementia brought to her mother, Doris. A graduate of the Columbia School of Social Work and married fifty years to Banesh Hoffmann, a colleague of Albert Einstein, Doris was a proud intellectual. When she was diagnosed at age eighty-four with an incurable disease of the mind, even though she had been having memory problems for fifteen years, it was an incredible blow. This was not Deborah's image of her mother; it was beneath her.

Deborah says the first time Doris asked how they were related, it knocked her breath away. Then there was the first time she asked if Deborah had been to New York, where she had lived for twenty-five years. And when had she first met Banesh? After enough times, however, Deborah wasn't upset anymore. And since the confusion didn't upset Doris, they took it in stride.

At a certain point Deborah stopped correcting, stopped insisting on the importance of reality, and that made it easier on her mother. And it liberated Deborah just to let it go by. It wasn't a big deal if it wasn't really April or they weren't really sorority sisters. Doris still thought Deborah was someone she cared a lot about and was happy to be with. It no longer even mattered that her daughter was gay; it was simply that she had a friend who made her happy, whom Doris also enjoyed. And then came Deborah's awakening: holding on to roles and images was the root of her suffering.

Deborah, who is now fifty, oversaw her mother's well-being for about five years, but as the situation unraveled it became more difficult, and ultimately impossible, to let her live alone. She hired some home aides for about a year for four hours a day, then six, eight, twelve—but Doris wasn't willing to let anyone stay in the apartment overnight. Then it simply wasn't safe anymore, so Deborah found a good residential care facility close by.

> All of the literature, the personal stories about Alzheimer's, they all refer to the devastation. And I agree. But they also refer to a person's loss of humanity, and I just don't agree. Even though my mother has very little recollection of the past, I don't believe that translates into a loss of humanity. It is shocking to us who rely on memories of the past, but she is truly, truly living in the moment, the ultimate enlightened person. I sense her spirit and her personality very much there. Sometimes someone will be sitting next to her, worse off than her, no verbal ability left, and my mother, who had never been particularly affectionate, is holding her hand, stroking her hair and face. How could you possibly say that's a person with no humanity? We have to separate out what *we're* going through from what the person we're caring for is going through.
>
> I'm very attached to my childhood memories; they tell me who I am. But it's clear to me you can still be somebody without it; you still have definition without a past. What is most difficult for people is they are no longer linked to the past the way you are, and so they're not linked to *you* in the way you want them to be and the way you're linked to them. I would be thrilled if she remembered that I'm her daughter, but it's not a loss to her. It's a loss to me.

Transcendence

About five years ago, Alan's father, Norman, began to succumb to the debilitating effects of Parkinson's disease. Alan's brother, John, was the main caregiver, but Alan was active with emotional and spiritual support. A choreographer and motivational speaker who relies heavily on intuition, Alan says that caring for his father propelled him into a deeper self-examination that has nourished both his creativity and sense of the sacred.

Norman was a quiet man, but he had a presence. Alan noticed that with the disease's progression, his father would focus intensely on every word, which tended to put Alan into a time shift, as if there were significance to each syllable. This meditative pace would stay with him in the workaday world, where he found himself listening more deeply to others, gaining "a soft heart for people who speak a lot with silence," he says.

Alan seemed to take on the role of reflecting back to his father his presence in the world, often in poetic frame. He borrowed from his own teaching techniques to help Norman come alive when he couldn't talk or was low in energy; gradually Alan realized *he* was the one receiving instruction in how to just hang out with a father.

> The greatest times were saying a few words, doing some work, reading. Dad was like a Zen roshi: inscrutable. Words weren't his deal anymore, but the right word would drop at the right time. He was educating us. He had tears in his eyes and I said to him, "You're really a graceful man, you're showing us how to die just like you showed us how to drive a car, or why we got an erection, or how to leave home for college." He was a very centered person; at the end of life he just got more quiet, bringing you back to the center even more just because of his presence. Whatever was bull's-eye in Dad all along, he kept to it but magnified it.

Forty-seven today, Alan honors caregiving as humbling, opening, saturating. He says he's gone through entire worlds of being transformed by the grace of sharing a parent's dying.

It comes on so gradually, like the way a shadow comes over a building, the way the light changes. It's like you have this secret knowledge that future caregivers' entire opinion of life will change. It bends you at first—I'm in the "responsible parent" role now with my daughter—and it's almost a revelation that you could take on that kind of adulthood.

Initially, there's this spiritual pinch of continually having to be patient and humble and suffer another indignity, and then this ridiculous complexity of paperwork that is like a frozen maiden in your house that seems to be uncaring. With elder care you may find out how to work the system, but it's an all-encompassing, overwhelming deal; you just want to go to the beach when it's over. Caregiving is an entire world, it's an entire engagement. Once you go through it, it's so spiritually transforming, it's very important to have some kind of closure.

Near the end it gets very mysterious, very intimate. It's such a big process. It's a walk into what you thought was a dark and unfamiliar land, but you find out it's your living room. You find out it's in between picking up your kid from school and going to work the next morning, and it fits in your life with your little benchmarks, and you're watching yourself grumble about it and he's got a week to live and what are you going to do after Dad dies and it's a relief to him. There's this poignant kind of humor to it: it's a very normal set of events at the human level.

Every moment you're alive, you've basically got the secret. So you see people getting pissed off and impatient, and there are people sitting in hospital beds wondering what the meaning of it all is; and this is like a flutter of wings past, and you realize you have only a few moments here. You will have frustrating times like money and traffic jams and who's respecting you, but if you're not established in the poignancy of the gift of being here, then you really miss the boat. It's a privilege to know that life has a big trick to play on you. In your last days, you see it really was a few moments; and if you had been more aware and conscious, you could have enjoyed a lot of them. This death story for my mid-forties is probably the greatest gift I could have gotten, to love and bless your life.

Living and dying are very related; they lead back to the center. Someone who has lost someone has gone on a first-person blind hero's journey, following his instincts so that he is happening to the world, rather than being a victim where the world is happening to him. This person has the license and the authority of righteousness to live a graceful life, to make it any way he wants at the end.

"In undertaking a spiritual life," writes Jack Kornfield, "what matters is simple: we must make certain that our path is connected with our heart." Then, with undivided intent, whatever we encounter is our spiritual practice.

In Buddhist lore the bodhisattva—having become enlightened—is the epitome of compassion, the awakened one who has turned from self-absorption to helping others. It is not that he does not suffer—he does—but his engagement in the world is voluntary. He is joyful because he lives in the present, mindful of all of life. No longer at the mercy of convention, no longer drawn to the goods of this world nor alarmed by mankind's condition, he is one with all that is, though not attached to it. Transcending desire, he has become liberated. Compassion is spirit made flesh.

Thank You for Everything

In my dream, people are milling about the pews of a funeral home. Someone is giving a eulogy, but I can't hear because a woman and her daughter are chatting disrespectfully several seats away. I go to hush them, but as I do, I glance over at Mother's black-draped coffin. Father is sitting there—youthful, radiant, tossing his head back and laughing impishly as he rocks back and forth, clasping his bent knees to his chest—on top of his wife's casket.

My aunt had suggested I not call Father on Thanksgiving as he was in so much pain and needed rest. I called anyway, needing to make contact. He was weak but thrilled. He told me about a ball game he had been watching and read me part of an article from the *Wall Street Journal*. I was happy to share his philosophy of sportsmanship and his opinions about the news, delighting in his lucidity until he said he was on a plane to Chicago.

Eventually, feeling I should get back to work, I asked him to give my love to Mother. He replied, "I will proffer it to her gently and sweetly." Those were the last words my father spoke to me.

He died that night, right in the middle of our turkey dinner, in bed-rattling pain. He asked Jennifer, the Arcadia director who had adopted my parents, to watch out for his Elaine, and she whispered that of course she would. Then he could let go. I told my boss I did not know when I would be back and left to find out what it meant to lose my father. Life hangs in the balance—and lives in love.

In a raging ice storm Bob and I headed straight for Mother. We found her alone, in her tangerine corduroy chair next to Dad's empty bed, sitting like a distracted little girl, legs crossed but restless, waiting, waiting for someone or something familiar. She looked up, startled, not understanding why we had come though the staff had told her. I could not fathom the agony Father must have been in to have had to leave his wife in this condition. Jennifer said that even in his final agonies, he was a consummate gentleman, continuing to stammer please and thank you.

The staff had fussed over Mother, who looked so small, so

innocent. Her question became obsessive: Where is Mel? And so I told her, over and over, each time a startling revelation, each time a stab in the heart as I kept killing my mother with the horrid truth, because she kept asking. Her anguish flowed in my veins.

We moved Mother to a semiprivate room in Arcadia, which pleased her friends there. At the condo we sorted belongings. While I was sifting through her dressers, a Proustian evocation slipped over me as the scent of her sweet perfumes lifted out of those drawers. I fixated on my mother's lingerie, on my father's suits, the intimate and personal effects, each with so many wonderful stories to tell: his top hat, still in the original 1940s box; the ties sent to New York to be laundered, still in their return boxes. I remained in their bedroom for hours, caressing everything as if to absorb my parents' presence and how truly safe they always made me feel.

Coincidentally, all funds ran out two days before Dad passed away. We decided to sell the Steinway, my sister relinquishing her inheritance to a higher purpose. When the piano man came by to make an offer, Bob and I went downstairs to thumb through our feelings. Marty began to tinker with scales, erupting into a beautiful classic. Everything clicked: the only possible legacy for my mother's most cherished possession was that it be played and enjoyed. And so we sold it, without her knowledge that the treasure that had sustained her in life would now keep her safe until death. Unable to watch, I left the house when the movers disassembled my mother's sixty years of inspiration. But we had enough money for one hundred days in the nursing home, and it was not possible, now that we knew death was real, that she could live so long. On the fiftieth anniversary of the bombing of Pearl Harbor, I secured my mother's safety.

One day I found a stuffed white unicorn at the foot of Mother's bed. No one knew how it had gotten there. She indicated with a tiny point that she wanted to hold it, so I placed it in her arms. As she willed some unknown strength to bring it to her emaciated breast, her tears spilled over its face. She covered it with kisses and gently stroked its fur. We sat for some time, uninterrupted, as she petted the animal and I petted her. I understood then that she had always known what had happened to her—and had borne it silently.

CHAPTER 15

The Urge to Serve

The characteristics of the man . . . under the rule of matter are fear, individualism, competition, and greed. These have to give place to spiritual confidence, co-operation, group awareness, and selflessness.—Alice A. Bailey, *The Labours of Hercules*

"There is hope in men—not in society, not in systems, organized religious systems, but in you and in me," said Krishnamurti. "Ultimately we shall be transformed, ultimately we shall be happy, ultimately we shall find truth. . . . Where love is, there is transformation . . . because love is transformation from moment to moment." Family caregiving is like this: love arises from service; service has come from love. Out of this subtle exchange comes new purpose in a timeless convergence of all that we have learned and become. Caregiving magnifies and focuses the best we have to offer, and gives us permission to live an authentic life—who we are at heart rather than who we think we should be. Our urge to care has become who we truly are.

From where does this mandate arise? Psychologist and scholar James Hillman believes that each of us has a calling, a *daimon* or destiny, the impression that there is a purpose we are born to fulfill and that we are guided from within to manifest it. It is not so much a matter of predisposed greatness but of character, which "forms a life regardless of how obscurely that life is lived and how little light falls on it from the stars. Calling becomes a calling to life . . . to honesty rather than to success, to caring and mating, to service and struggle for the sake of living."

The myth of the twelve labors of Hercules exemplifies this evolution. He is a reminder of what lives within all of us: the ability to overcome obstacles in order to generate what has real meaning and vitality. Hercules pledges himself to divine will, rounding the zodiac until fear and pride are banished and perfection emerges. Life is redreamed: welcoming a world of sorrow, we are released from sorrow; in service, we find our destiny.

For many caregivers, the vision of suffering catalyzes an urge to help relieve it. Life becomes devotional practice, not out of duty but from great good joy.

An Advocate for Caregivers

Caregiving consecrates life by nurturing a person's ability to reach out. But how do we offer a boon to the world that doesn't recognize its own need? One answer is to keep trying, until small responses form a larger voice. Suzanne Mintz is cofounder and president of the National Family Caregivers Association (NFCA), headquartered near Washington, D.C. A tireless advocate for visibility and respect for family caregiving, her life was interrupted almost twenty-five years ago when she was just twenty-eight: she learned that her husband of seven years, Steven, then thirty-one, had multiple sclerosis (MS).

Outwardly their lives didn't change much, but nothing was the same. Suzanne was apprehensive about almost everything, uncertain how to communicate with Steven about his feelings and needs. He turned inward for strength; she sought outer support to feel she wasn't alone in coping. They confided in family, but difficulties mounted until the couple separated—two times, once for two years before reconciliation.

Suzanne channeled her frustrations into a drive for success but ended up in a psychiatrist's office, paralyzed by clinical depression. There, for the first time, she let herself cry. When she emerged from the turmoil, she decided to refocus on a broader goal: to help other family caregivers. With her pal Cindy Fowler, a graphic designer whose mother had Parkinson's disease, they founded NFCA with an eye to improving the overall quality of life for caregivers.

As Steven's MS has progressed, so has Suzanne's crusade.

We don't suggest that giving care is as hard as needing it. But the caregiver gives up dreams, too. Becoming a caregiver means re-evaluating priorities, making compromises, spending thousands of dollars on equipment your insurance doesn't cover. Caregiving is learning about drugs and emergency-alert systems. It's hard work and pain—and joy when your loved one has a good day. And yet there is a total loss of normalcy: the things the rest of the world takes for granted are things that trouble caregivers every day.

With great empathy and a desire to make a difference, Suzanne left her marketing job in one of the nation's top architectural firms to become a full-time advocate. To that end, NFCA has created a peer support network, a speakers bureau, and a newsletter and actively promotes National Family Caregivers Week each November. The organization has commissioned a large caregiver survey, published an extensive resource guide, and procured sponsorship from pharmaceuticals and health product manufacturers to promote caregiver health and public awareness. Suzanne also lobbied to have caregivers counted as a category in the census—not only to urge them to recognize themselves, but also to mobilize service providers, policy makers, and researchers.

This is not just a personal issue to be dealt with only within the confines of our families, but rather a social issue that must be addressed. Illness and disability are a family affair, and caregivers are at risk themselves. If we are given more support and education, we will feel more empowered, have more satisfaction and pride in ourselves, and that in turn will make us more effective caregivers. The impact of a global aging population is at the tip of these issues. Medical technology has been wonderful at keeping people alive a lot longer than they would have lived, but we have not looked into the consequences of that and the impact it has on families—not just extending life, but quality of life.

Fighting for Research

Moral concerns propel many people into national and global arenas when their caregiving days are over. It is no longer enough to have done a good job and then to return to business as usual. For many, there is no such thing: life is different now and so is its purpose.

Carol Walton, fifty-three, has taken her cause all the way to Capitol Hill in the years since she was a long-distance caregiver to her father, who died of Parkinson's disease a few years ago. She not only battled her own ignorance and fear but also her father's denial. He would not eat well or exercise, wouldn't take the right medications, was losing his balance and falling. Everything was happening at once, leaving Carol at wits' end.

Over seven painstaking years, she learned by trial and error how to use social services and how to find new housing as the disease progressed because facilities weren't geared to his level of disability. Networking from a couple of states away was aggravating. She had to move her father five times to different levels of assisted living, because of both the progression of the disease and her lack of awareness of long-term planning. Although her father probably should have been admitted to a higher level of care much earlier, she and her brother, who shared some of the responsibilities, simply didn't understand.

At one point her father, three years from death, was yanking out his feeding tube. Either his hands had to be wrapped so he couldn't continue or someone had to spend ten hours a day at bedside to restrain him. Nursing care from temporary agencies was inconsistent at best; each person had to be educated about stomach feeding. Eventually Carol hired a nurse, at great expense, just to watch her father around the clock. Then he was found wandering on the freeway. Carol thought, "This just isn't working."

She didn't know a lot of things back then: how to care for him and make him happy, how to spend hard time at the convalescent facility when other family members wouldn't. But she did the best she could, even though her father treated her and her brother badly. People asked how she could bear it, but she knew he was mad at the whole world. It wasn't personal. She also discovered that she needed to be at the facility every shift, meeting nurses and assistants, networking and bringing them doughnuts and coffee, finding out what they did for her father and how he was doing because he was mum.

After it was over, Carol was left with a burning desire to push for changes in health care and for research on a disease that costs an estimated $25 billion annually. Her understanding of what caregiving families go through and the bewilderment of dealing with difficult behaviors led her to form a consumer action network and to organize caregiver education and leadership training. Then she moved into the congressional arena, gathering sponsorship for the Morris K. Udall Parkinson's Research and Education Act that authorized a fourfold increase in spending at the National Institutes of Health—$100 million a year for four to five years. The measure passed; now she is working on the appropriations segment.

Carol has also organized representatives of the four major Parkinson's groups into a single task force with a unified agenda. In tirelessly pursuing her cause, she has discovered a gift for combining her consulting background with an eye to revealing the forgotten elderly in modern society. She does a lot of volunteer work, gives workshops and training seminars, and has adopted several elders in a nearby convalescent home whom she visits regularly.

Says Carol, "So many powerful, positive things have come out of this experience; it's rare to think back now about how bad it was. Some people never understand what their gifts are and how to use them. But everything in life happens for a reason. I didn't believe that my father had this disease for twelve years for nothing, but it was for me to figure it out, to honor it."

Nothing Is Impossible

Classical spiritual tenets teach that without sacrifice, there is no spiritual enlightenment. For actress and film director Elizabeth Sung, the passion to help others grew out of the loss of her brother to AIDS at age twenty-six. He had been her inspiration and support in the worst of times, her greatest fan in the best of times. She cared for Philip when AIDS in the Asian community, let alone in mainstream America and Europe, was a hushed affair—and long before AIDS in Africa and Asia started making headlines.

Elizabeth emigrated from Hong Kong to the United States in 1973 with the dream of becoming a professional ballet dancer. Educated in a convent, she had begun studying dance at age five. But her father, a political activist and entrepreneur, was opposed to careers in the arts for his children. However, after he passed away, she and her sister, Diana, went to New York and joined their brother, Philip, who was pursuing a career in fashion design and already had his own company after graduating from the Fashion Institute of Technology on Hong Kong's first scholarship.

Philip inspired Elizabeth to follow her heart. He was both brother and surrogate father; he looked out for her and provided for her college education. She was accepted into the prestigious Juilliard School, then joined the Alvin Ailey national touring company. After a debilitating back injury crippled her dance career, she studied acting with Sanford Meisner and at Uta Hagen's HB studio. Then her brother was diagnosed with the disease.

Elizabeth shelved her ambitions for two years to care for him, taking a job in an import company just to secure an income. Meanwhile, caregiving gave her time to think about the meaning of life. "Philip was my role model for pursuing, unwaveringly, what he loved to do. Looking at him, it flooded my mind that I had never given myself a chance. Especially after he got ill, he talked to me of the concept of transformation, what an artistic life means. He said that if we pick that road, we cannot just live and expect immediate gratification—it's a lifelong commitment and ultimately, with passion and love, I will break away from a sense of limitation to a higher place."

Elizabeth was sickened by the lack of support for those suffering with AIDS and by the stigma and condemnation attached to the disease. Even today, she says, there is still strong denial worldwide; people continue to think they are invincible or that AIDS will not infect them. There is also an awkwardness between generations that makes breaking the news so fearful, so most choose to keep the truth hidden. She was tormented by how families abandon sons with AIDS and especially by how it struck her brother when he was so young and everything was going well.

The lack of caring in society and the world added to the difficulty in making peace with the situation. As a caregiver Elizabeth experienced what so many have in the AIDS pandemic: the ostracism of those infected extends to their caretakers; everywhere there is guilt, shame, and feelings of inadequacy. Not only are grief and fear of pain and loss ever present—and usually with multiple losses, as in the gay community—but not much mental health support exists for burnout and compassion fatigue. Although HIV has infected intravenous drug users, blood bank recipients, older people, heterosexual men and women, and even newborns, and although research has seen the disease lose its status as an automatic death sentence, still it is perceived less compassionately than cancer or Alzheimer's.

But these challenges gave Elizabeth resilience and determination. She thought about all the things Philip had taught her about life, and after a period of introspection and piercing sorrow, she again looked to the creative arts. She landed television roles and a part in Wayne Wang's film *The Joy Luck Club* and then on CBS's top daytime soap, *The Young and the Restless*. Meanwhile she married Philip Tulipan, a fellow actor and screenwriter she had met while at the HB studio.

Although Elizabeth was trapped in sadness for some time, she realized she had the choice to turn around an impossible situation and allow it instead to be a source of strength and focus. She had thought about being a director but never let herself fantasize too much. Then, having faced losing a loved one and seeing how quickly life goes by, "it was a wake-up call—that if you love something, you can't procrastinate. It was a catalytic moment and gave me the strength to go toward acting and then evolve into directing."

She was one of twelve—out of four hundred applicants among industry professionals—selected for the American Film Institute's (AFI) Directing Workshop for Women. Her assignment was to create a half-hour drama. She looked within to see what she would like to share and decided to pay tribute to her brother. She sat down with her husband

and outlined her story, recounting twenty years in America. She wanted to tell about a brother-sister relationship and to use the film as an opportunity to bring to light the humanity in us all.

Requiem, Elizabeth's story of loss and hope, was featured in film festivals and fund-raising events. Among its many honors were the CINE Golden Eagle and Distinguished Filmmaker Award from New Horizon Artworks; it was the highlight of a screening at the Academy of Television Arts and Sciences in Los Angeles, a benefit for the Asian Pacific AIDS Intervention Team. Its success was another turning point. "If I wanted to be an artist, I could not just hope that I would have all the equipment. I needed to be willing to accept change. Even though something tragic happened, some of the restrictive part of me died and a new me was born out of that process. My brother's message of transformation was letting go of pain even though you're embedded with it when someone dear to you dies—to not be the victim of a mournful situation. You have to believe in your calling and the right to go after it."

Elizabeth has completed her second-year AFI thesis, *The Water-Ghost*, about a young girl who lost her mother and stopped living because of sadness. The story line's thread is deliberate: the continuation of her journey of losing a loved one, and her desire to give a voice to immigrant women.

Once you're strong and allow yourself to do all the things you love, you can help other people either directly or indirectly as a source of encouragement. If you have the chance to share your story, you can encourage them to move beyond the point of tragedy.

Nobody deserves to die in shame. There is nothing more important than letting people know they are loved and have lived a meaningful life. The caregiving journey is like being reborn again and again and again because when you are taking care of someone you are like a guardian soldier, doing what they are not able to do. In a short time you become strong beyond what you are usually capable of doing. Out of those experiences you see life and death are a part of the process of life; there is always a beginning and an ending, and there is an added layer of knowingness, of acceptance. Nothing is impossible except fear. There is no limit to each and every one of us. Life is about giving.

The Art of Caring for Others

Each life cycle is an initiation into broader relationship with the world. For one woman who cofounded three major Alzheimer's organizations, each passage has marked a notch in her lifelong crusade to help relieve suffering and to build a strong community of people who take care of each other.

Anne Bashkiroff's mandate grew out of years of torturous necessity—what she calls a cross between *Dr. Zhivago* and *One Flew over the Cuckoo's Nest.* The saga of the woman who pioneered advocacy for those with brain impairments more than twenty years ago began with a young girl's passion for a man who was the epitome of intelligence, charm, and class. Alexander ("Sasha") Bashkiroff was twenty years older than Anne, but their common heritage was a deep bond. He came from great wealth in pre-Revolutionary Russia—he was raised by governesses and maids, and his early memories were of jewels and furs and mansions decorated by foreign architects and landscaped by botanists. But after the Bolshevik Revolution in 1917, Sasha had to find a livelihood, so he went east and earned degrees in electrical and mechanical engineering from a polytechnic institute in Manchuria.

In the same period Anne's family fled from the Ukraine to Siberia, where Jews were not persecuted, and then on to China, where she was born and raised. Although she has wonderful memories of her childhood there, she was without a country and yearned for stability. When Anne was only fifteen she met Sasha in Shanghai; he managed a swank apartment complex nearby. They went their own ways during the Japanese occupation of Shanghai and World War II; at twenty, she saw him at a party and they began dating. But the political situation was explosive, and Anne immigrated to the United States with her mother. Sasha followed six months later. They married on Independence Day in 1947, believing that America was God's country, where hopes could be fulfilled.

Inseparable, for twenty years they lived out the American dream, raising a son and enjoying work and friends. But then Sasha became ill with a serious fever and needed a kidney operation. It was the beginning of an endless tunnel. At sixty-five, Sasha suddenly lacked the vigor or interest in working that had characterized his life. He tried to work but was fired for forgetting instructions. So Anne became the breadwinner, not a role she had been raised to assume. They bounced from doctor to doctor; after a dozen of them, one neurologist declared Sasha's problem to be presenile dementia.

In the beginning it's the denial, she says of the fearfulness and isolation. "I don't remember what else transpired. I rushed out of the office, grabbed my husband's arm, and ran. And that is what I kept doing for the next six years—running. Running from physicians who told me he had irreversible brain damage, from friends who tried to tell me there was something strange about my husband, from myself, from life itself."

Mixed together were tremendous love and tremendous pity for this person whom she loved so much and who was being destroyed. Because dementia was not socially acceptable, she felt as if her entire family were tainted. Friends, embarrassed for the couple, vanished. In the public arena it wasn't much easier. In order to find help, she had to stay home from work and call agency after agency for advice; nobody knew what to tell her. Anne also had to devise ways to keep Sasha occupied at home while she worked; while she tried to sleep, he wandered or unhooked pipes. She would discover the kitchen floor inundated with water in the middle of the night.

Soon her mother and father also became dependent: at one time all three of them were hospitalized on the same floor and she could hear them calling to her from different rooms, needy and upset, splitting her into so many pieces that she came apart. "No matter how much you love the person, there isn't enough of you to go around. You are absolutely emptied out, and when your energy goes, you have nothing left. Nobody must be asked to martyr their lives; this is not right."

For seven years Anne kept Sasha at home, witness to the progressive attrition she was powerless to prevent. She thought she could cope, but her identity was wrapped up in being Sasha's wife. As he slid down the precipice, she had nothing to hold on to. Their son was a teenage boy and needed his mother, but Anne was strained past her limits because her husband was also like a child. At one point she even contemplated suicide. "I felt imprisoned by Sasha's disease," she says. "I was completely enveloped in it, from dressing him, feeding him, making sure he didn't wander, to cleaning up after him when he lost control of his bodily functions. I never stopped loving him, but exhaustion overtook love and became the predominant emotion."

As the dementia progressed, it became clear that Anne could no longer care for Sasha because he needed twenty-four-hour help. He had become confused and belligerent, a danger to himself. But where could she place him? There were no facilities in those days handling such problems. Costs for convalescence were considerable: nearly $1,000 a month for custodial care not covered by the couple's comprehensive major-medical policy, a financial tsunami that Anne didn't know about ahead of time.

Sasha was thrown out of eight places in three months, sometimes within an hour of arrival. Three times he escaped; he was returned to the psychiatric hospital where he had been placed before, which Anne hated for him. Their insurance covered limited treatment for aggressive behavior, but then she had to find him a permanent home. They were middle income: too rich to qualify for welfare, too poor to survive the strain of massive long-term bills. Anne and Sasha hadn't immigrated in order to collect taxpayer dollars. "When we came to this country, it was impressed upon us that we must have enough money so we would not become public charges. To me it is an irony beyond description that the system now says, 'We're not going to help you until you become a public charge.'"

But a miracle occurred: thirty women board members of Children's Hospital, where Anne worked, took up a collection to help her out monthly. She was overcome with gratitude and promised the debt would be repaid.

Eventually Sasha was placed in a skilled nursing facility. He had become totally withdrawn and didn't recognize Anne or his twenty-three-year-old son. He had aged a million years in those few months, Anne says. The seeds had been sown for her outrage over the lack of care and compassion for those with irreversible brain damage. Tenacious in her new mandate, Anne became part of the San Francisco Mental Health Association's Family Survival Task Force and overcame shyness to speak before then First Lady Rosalynn Carter at the President's Commission on Mental Health. Anne pleaded for understanding for brain-impaired patients, for dignity, for attention to the lack of facilities and the astronomical costs for long-term custodial care. It was the beginning of a mission that resulted, among other accomplishments, in formation of the Family Survival Project, which became Family Caregiver Alliance, today a statewide resource agency and powerhouse network on the World Wide Web.

Ironically, the day that the California Legislature granted state funds for the caregiver agency, Sasha died, among strangers in a facility guarded by a seven-foot-high wire fence. His wife and son were two hours away.

Anne's hard work also resulted in her cofounding the Alzheimer's Association and its offspring, the Alzheimer's Disease and Related Disorders Association. They have become global influences in research and support for diseases that steal the mind. But her crusade has also been a catharsis: doing for others reclaimed her life and set her on a path of joyful service.

> You become a nonperson through all this. I had to reestablish myself as a human being—the loss of a husband is a loss of identity because he is part of you. We need each other, and we need to help each other. As we say in Russia, "We all walk under God." Nobody has the luxury of not paying attention to this—they don't know what's waiting for them tomorrow. Helping other people is what got me out of the depression. My character has withstood a storm and has been polished by it. When I married Sasha I was judgmental, impatient, and held flimsy interpretations of life. Now compassion has become an integral part of my character. I cannot listen to the problems of others without the reaction of, "What can I do?" My life has changed irrevocably and upward for joy because of what I went through. As much as we want only happiness as kids and teens, that's terrific; but unless you've suffered in your life you really don't know what happiness is.

Anne, who continues the campaign for public awareness in her seventies, says she recognized that she always had a choice either to say she did the best she could and move on or to extend a hand back. She couldn't walk away. "I was so filled with the feeling that I could not be the only one going through this, there had to be others, and the only reason nothing is being done is because no one has spoken out, people aren't aware of the problems. I have always believed that people would care. Even though no one can do this all by themselves, each of us has the power together."

At the end of a biography by Gail Bernice Holland, *For Sasha with Love*, Anne concludes: "If there is to be any meaning to my life—and to Sasha's life—and if there is to be any meaning to the inherent promises Sasha and I treasured as immigrants entering America, then it has to lie in the ultimate art of caring for one another."

Because caregivers have touched both poles—suffering and generosity—they are given a vision of the whole, the world beyond self. Helping others can become a calling from the far side of grief, a mandate to assuage psycho-spiritual ghosts that remain long after the physical tasks have been accomplished—or even in the midst of them. Those who are touched by compassion discover life at its purest, honoring the mystery of service and the value of each person.

"The highest service we can perform is to assist that process [of manifesting wholeness] within ourselves, within others and within the world. . . . Revelation is not a great Being telling man what to do. It is his own being seeking to release itself," writes visionary David Spangler in *Revelation*.

Family caregiving is a wrenching, humbling experience for those who venture all the way in. Once the heart is open, it does not fail to see suffering all around. But in gratefulness for the truth about life and death, it is capable of sustaining lovingkindness. To replace self-love with service is to begin the transformation of more than just the individual. The secrets of the soul are revealed to those who care.

Our Love Will Never End

After three weeks of attending to Mother and estate matters, there was nothing more to be done. Bob and I needed to return to our jobs and a sense of a normal life, so we decided to drive back to California and wait for word. One last evening we sat in the nursing home's activities room, listening to classical music as Mom's fingers marked constricted phrases in her lap. For the first time I broke down in her presence, confessing so much regret about what had befallen them, how much I adored them. She understood. With a slight tilt of her head she directed us to a pink balloon on the bookshelf. She wanted to play a game, and so Bob and his second mother batted it around with their heads, the two as one as we three became one, without a care in the world, back and forth. Time stopped, and we had music and moments enough to love.

Then Mother and I sat face to face. She crawled her fingers over to my knee to touch it, to take my hand to her lap, her hands on either side, patting me, gazing into me. In that moment we were connected in eternity. She was Everymother, the nurturing feminine, telegraphing a message to sustain me long after she was gone. Then dinner arrived and it was time for us to leave. Mother pierced me with a look: we two were everything, all the life that had ever lived, all the love that had ever loved. Bob and I walked to the door and waved, smiling, and she acknowledged us with a grin. Then she turned to the meal and vanished into her world. I never saw my mother again.

A week later, on my forty-third birthday, I phoned the nursing station to have them fetch Mother. I could hear her shuffling down the hall, and when I spoke to her, she only grunted, and then left the phone dangling. Shortly afterward she stopped eating. Jennifer, director and friend, reported that Mother had indicated she was starving on purpose; she wanted to be with her husband. Shortly after the new year it was over. She didn't choke, she didn't suffer; she died in peace of her own conscious will, weighing only fifty pounds and too weak even to tear a piece of Kleenex. She let go in full knowledge that she was loved and that she had loved deeply.

Even though I was grateful for the mercy, losing my mother was even harder than losing my father. For a daughter, a father's passing is like missing a beloved piece of ourselves that attaches after birth, but a mother's death disconnects us from the source of life itself. Now that she was gone, I was an orphan. Never again would I share in my parents' love and guidance. At her funeral we played the videotape of her last piano concert—when she was already stricken but no one knew it—and the congregation understood, finally, the muse that had inhabited her all those years. Even in death she brought tears of joy through her music. She was buried in the dead of winter as her coffin was lowered into three feet of icy water and rain fell like applause.

Bob and I left Wichita in a sleet storm to drive back to California. We closed the condo; we visited the grave site. No words could touch the depth of my sorrow; I did not know what was inside my heart. Their suffering was so unfair, but it was never meaningless. The knowledge that my parents were out of pain meant that my own healing could begin.

In June I held the ceremony to unveil the headstone at their grave site. On the spur of the moment I returned to the condominium one last time, before the bank foreclosed because of unresolvable business debts. As I drifted through remembrances in each room, I heard an unfamiliar sound from the deck, a long song, rich and deep, billowing in crescendos and diminuendos. I thought, "No, it couldn't be, not after all these years." I sneaked to the back door, and it was: two cardinals, one scarlet and the other tan, chirping insistently at me. The female flew off but the male stayed for more than two hours, warbling in the large tree above me, unafraid. These had always been my parents' signature birds and had even appeared in Aunt Sam's dreams; but never in fifteen years had I seen any at the condo. I cried for joy, an unshakable impression that I wasn't alone—that love is eternal.

A month later I had this dream:

> I am sitting with my parents at a table in a movie theater lobby. My father keeps repeating a phrase, his eyes teasing. Finally it registers: "The red cardinal only comes out in the winter." He says it over and over until its full force hits me. I jump up: "So it *was* you at the condo!" My parents kick back their heads, roaring and laughing yes, yes, and I run to them and we hug until I wake up.

CHAPTER 16

Caregiving and Community

We know that every moment is a moment of grace, every hour an offering; not to share them would be to betray them. Our lives no longer belong to us alone; they belong to all who need us desperately.—Elie Wiesel, Nobel Peace Prize acceptance speech

As I am writing tonight, two preteens have gunned down several classmates; a disgruntled employee has killed two supervisors; a mother is suspected of smothering her three babies. We may think these horrors happen only "out there," but they are in fact part of each of us. The killing grounds have been created out of partial lives and isolation, out of the culture of complaint we take as real. There *is* a breakdown of connection and community. But the way of violence is not all that we are.

Caught up in a communication smog that soaks us in images of crime and hatred, we think we have little power for change. But there are no insignificant acts of benevolence. Each adds to the force of good in the world and impels humanity toward conscious evolution. I submit that family caregivers are proof that we are, all of us, much more capable of goodness than we imagined: not by random acts of kindness but by very deliberate ones, thoughtful and consistent and true.

Every day in tens—probably hundreds—of millions of homes around the world, frail elders and disabled spouses and children are receiving love and tenderness. Every day family members, friends, neighbors, and service professionals do great good to assuage illness, grief, and untold loss. These commonplace actions do not garner headlines, but they are far more prevalent than evil. They are acts that defy death even though death is the inevitable conclusion; in the face of uncertainty, love prevails. The heart is alive and well, and it abides.

We say we want to live forever, but we also want to remain young. In this duplicity we prefer to quarantine the elderly lest they remind us of what can be taken away—ignoring the fact that more older people are healthy and active than ever before and will be even more so. Ageism in fact may be the only "ism" still socially acceptable. Our compartmentalization of old age is arbitrary, our ignorance of what it means to be fully alive alarming. With a tidal wave of demographics upon us, we can no longer afford to ignore what later life might be saying.

Paranoia and bias must be given up now. Old age is not a competition, a medical problem to be conquered, but a life passage to be honored and integrated. In addressing the core values around aging and death, we see that we do not mature from cradle to grave, but wisdom is handed back in the other direction. And each person adds to its power.

"The nature of aging has to do with change," says Ram Dass. "The art of being able to look directly at death, and directly at suffering, is a function of your ability to find in yourself that which is not changing. That's spiritual work; that's the journey of aging." That is also the journey of caregiving, which hones this ability to look directly at loss and to nurture what does not change. It reveals the stability of the human heart to remain open in the midst of trauma, to rest in the still point of the turning world, as poet T. S. Eliot said, anchored to the authority of its innate virtues.

In his quest to understand the ideas and beliefs that hold a society together, gerontologist Robert Kastenbaum has taken the study of aging into the realm of the spirit. His conclusions extend well beyond tradition and illuminate the heart of caregiving. He proposes that aging is not about how we grow old, but about what life means if our fate is to both age and die—that how we define old age, and what it should be, is one of society's most critical tests of strength.

Ultimately he believes the well-being of the elderly—and by extension, humanity itself—can be protected only by appreciating the intimate interdependence of life and respect for the whole person. "Limitations and distortions in our core vision of what it means to be a person become starkly evident in old age. If to be an old person is to suffer abandonment, disappointment and humiliation, this is not a 'geriatric problem.' It is the disproof of our whole shaky pudding, technology, science, and all. If our old people are empty, our vision of life is empty."

Aging and dying teach us that a person's greatest virtue is the capacity to give. If we really want to help in the world, we must learn how to live in it. And we cannot do that if we do not participate mindfully in all of it, just as it is. We are asked to pay attention to the untended business of life, to ameliorate the relationships we thought were formed and finished in our youth. We must recapitulate the habits and the identities created long ago that bind us to uniform behaviors hardened against the fluidity that life demands. Our value systems must reconnect the full spectrum of life.

Until we view aging as something other than suffering and loss to be avoided, we will continue to live with social institutions based on fear. Policy issues are immense, and people now at midlife will be ferrying them into the future. They center on whether family networks can continue to provide as much help in the future, when because of social trends more elders will be divorced, unmarried, or without children. Concerns will include how to maintain disabled elders in the community by:

~ Obtaining funding
~ Preventing disability
~ Increasing research funding for such ravages of late life as Alzheimer's, osteoporosis, and stroke

~ Promoting responsibility for more vital aging
~ Designing age-sensitive independent-living communities
~ Redefining old age to engage elders in their communities and workplaces as natural resources

There is movement; more attention *is* being paid to social and moral responsibility in schools, in businesses, and in health care. One hopeful indication of this shift is the Relationship-Centered Care Network. Composed of health care professionals and academic institutions, its aim is to integrate biomedical, psycho-social, and spiritual realms into medical practice. "Healer and sufferer are not separate and independent units," according to the Pew-Fetzer Task Force charged with implementing this new vision of health care. "The need for the health professions [for] contemplative disciplines calls for a profound change in professional education, from a curriculum dominated by abstractions . . . to one balanced between intellectual analysis and the depths of human experience." This quest demands authenticity and integrity; it requires that everyone learn how to listen, how to communicate, and how to respond with compassion. It is both the science and the art of caring. As one fourth-year medical student said, " 'Do Not Resuscitate' does not mean 'Do Not Care.' "

Where do we find the means to go beyond limited perceptions of how to care for each other and how to develop supports relevant to the new reality of older age? I believe that the key lies no farther than our own living rooms. Caregiving is about communion. It demands that we reestablish relationship at the center of our lives. When we take the time, we become aware of a truth that eluded us until we took this journey: we are not alone and need not be. Where love is exchanged, a triumphant connection is built to the guiding force in which we live and move and have our being.

When consciously carried forth, family caregiving offers the potential to discover the forgotten, lonely, and disparate parts of ourselves lost to our psyche's shadowland. It affords an opportunity to change the way we interact with everyone in each moment and from there to ameliorate life on earth. For if we have opened our hearts to suffering, we cannot ignore the world. The choice is ours in each moment whether to give or take, hate or love, act or recoil. It takes work; it takes sacrifice; most of all, it takes commitment. But if we are to turn the tide of this violent and reckless crisis point, the opportunity to do so lies right in our own homes. We do not even have to step outside to change the world.

"Love and compassion are necessities, not luxuries," says the Dalai Lama. If we are to evolve on this creaking planet so full of war and rage and starvation and homelessness, mankind must awaken. With a world on the cusp of change that will necessitate unfathomable levels of caring, it is not unreasonable to envision a way of being that is more aware of both suffering and service. We are at a threshold, a point of highest resistance that must synthesize into something greater than its opposing forces if it is to survive. Tensions and stakes are high: the status quo doesn't work anymore, neither in society nor in spirit. The curtain is rising to reveal that we must think globally. We can no longer equate independence with smug superiority.

It is not only acts of largesse that will carry humanity forward, however, but especially each spark of affection and thoughtfulness. It is the everyday people in their everyday roles who have gone a little farther than they thought they could, drummed up more audacity and heart than they believed possible. It is the support they give, an attentive and caring presence, that lays the foundation for advancement. "For it is not society that is to guide and save the creative hero, but precisely the reverse," wrote Joseph Campbell in *The Hero with a Thousand Faces*. "And so every one of us shares the supreme ordeal . . . not in the bright moments of his tribe's great victories, but in the silences of his personal despair."

For years I have listened to caregivers tell their stories, at first crying out for help from the nothingness that descended over them in a haze of despair. Then, as they have discovered the companionship of those who care, they have reached out to help others. It has been instinctive, it has been natural, but most of all it has been a deliberate mission to change "business as usual" in societies that have allowed aging and disability to be demonized.

One voice *can* make a difference; the sleeper must awaken. Where our hearts have opened, connections become automatic. For it is by tenacity that our spirits are carried forward; it is by sharing in the fortitude of others—by borrowing from it, if necessary, until it is our own—that we emerge from the battlefield stretched and bloodied, yet blessed and inspired.

The possibilities for caregiving to transform individuals and communities are limited only by our willingness to heed the call of those in need, to lose ourselves in service, to stand up and give voice to the suffering that is in our power to overcome. Depending upon our response, spiritual transformation is within reach. Depending on the love we bring forth, there is no longer anything to fear.

Walk softly

just awareness

the heart is open

Resources, Further Reading, Web Sites

Aging

Administration on Aging
330 Independence Ave., SW
Washington, DC 20201
(202) 619-0724
Directory of aging sites
www.aoa.dhhs.gov/aoa/webres/
craig.htm
Internet and E-Mail Resources on
Aging
www.aoa.dhhs.gov/aoa/pages/
jpostlst.html

Age Concern England
Astral House
1268 London Road
London SW16 4ER
England
www.ace.org.uk

American Association of Retired
Persons (AARP)
601 E St., NW
Washington, DC 20049
(202) 434-2277

(800) 424-3410
Fact sheets, booklets
www.aarp.org/caregive/home.htm
AARP Internet Resource Guide to
Aging
www.aarp.org/cyber/guide1/htm

Australia Council on the Aging
3 Bowen Crescent, Level 2
Melbourne, Victoria 3004
Australia
(03) 9820-2655
avoca.vicnet.net.au/~cotaa/

Canada Association for Retired
Persons (CARP)
27 Queen St. East, Suite 702
Toronto, Ontario M5C 2M6
Canada
(416) 363-5562

National Association for Hispanic
Elderly
234 E. Colorado Blvd., Suite 300
Pasadena, CA 91101
(626) 564-1988

National Caucus and Center on Black
Aged
1424 K St., NW, Suite 500
Washington, DC 20005
(202) 637-8400

National Council on the Aging
409 Third St., SW, Second Floor
Washington, DC 20024
(202) 479-1200
(800) 424-9046
www.ncoa.org

National Pacific/Asian Resource
Center on Aging
Melbourne Tower
1511 Third Ave., Suite 914
Seattle, WA 98101
(800) 336-2722

Further Reading

Mark E. Williams, *The American
Geriatric Society's Complete Guide to
Aging and Health.* New York:
Harmony Books, 1995.

Web Sites

American Geriatrics Society
www.americangeriatrics.org

American Society on Aging
www.asaging.org

ElderWeb
www.elderweb.com

National Institute on Aging Information Center
www.nih.gov/nia

Temple University Institute on Aging
www.temple.edu/aging/

Alternative Medicine

American Holistic Health Association
P.O. Box 17400
Anaheim, CA 92817-7400
(714) 779-6152
www.ahha.org

American Holistic Medical Association
6728 Old McLean Village Drive
McLean, VA 22101-3906
(703) 556-9728
www.ahmaholistic.org

Foundation for Integrative Medicine
(800) 523-3296
www.drweil.com

National Institutes of Health
Office of Alternative Medicine
888-644-6226

Directory of Alternative Healthcare
Associations
www.altmed.od.nih.gov

Preventive Medicine Research
Institute
Dr. Dean Ornish
900 Bridgeway, Suite 2
Sausalito, CA 94965
(415) 332-2525
(800) 328-3738

Stress Reduction Clinic
Dr. Jon Kabat-Zinn, Director
University of Massachusetts Medical
Center
Worcester, MA 01655
(508) 856-2656

The Wellness Community
2716 Ocean Park Blvd., Suite 1040
Santa Monica, CA 90405
(310) 314-2555

Further Reading

Jon Kabat-Zinn, *Full Catastrophe
Living: Using the Wisdom of Your
Body and Mind to Face Stress, Pain,
and Illness.* New York: Delacorte
Press, 1990.
Michael Lerner, *Choices in Healing:
Integrating the Best of Conventional
and Complementary Approaches to
Cancer.* Cambridge, MA: MIT
Press, 1994.

Christiane Northrup, *Women's Bodies, Women's Wisdom*. New York: Bantam, 1998.

Andrew Weil, *8 Weeks to Optimum Health*. New York: Fawcett Books, 1998.

Web Sites

The Alternative Medicine Homepage
www.pitt.edu/~cbw/altm.html

Chopra Center for Well Being
www.chopra.com

HealthWorld Online
www.healthy.net

Alzheimer's

Alzheimer's Association
Alzheimer's Disease and Related
   Disorders Association
919 N. Michigan Ave., Suite 1000
Chicago, IL 60611-1676
(312) 335-8700
(800) 272-3900
www.alz.org
Spirituality for caregivers
www.alz.org/lib/rlists/spirit.html
Stress and caregivers
www.alz.org/lib/rlists/stress.html

Alzheimer's Disease Education &
   Referral Center
P.O. Box 8250
Silver Spring, MD 20907-8250
(800) 438-4380
www.alzheimers.org/adear

Alzheimer's Disease International
45/46 Lower Marsh
London SE1 7RG
England
00 44 171 620 3011
www.alz.co.uk

Further Reading

Jo Danna, *When Alzheimer's Hits Home: Spotlight on a Public Health Crisis*. New York: Palomino Press, 1995.

Howard Gruetzner, *Alzheimer's: A Caregiver's Guide and Sourcebook*. New York: John Wiley & Sons, 1992.

Nancy Mace and Peter Rabins, *The 36-Hour Day: A Family Guide to Caring for Persons with Alzheimer's Disease, Related Dementia Illness and Memory Loss at Later Life*. Baltimore: Johns Hopkins University Press, 1991.

Mark Warner, *The Complete Guide to Alzheimer's-Proofing Your Home*. West Lafayette, IN: Purdue University Press, 1998.

Web Sites

Alzheimer's Association of Canada
www.alzheimer.ca

Alzheimer's Association/Europe
www.alzheimer-europe.org

Alzheimer's.com
www.alzheimers.com

Alzheimer's Disease Research Center/
   Northern Virginia
www.alz-nova.org

Alzheimer's Disease Society of the
   United Kingdom
www.vois.org.uk/alzheimers

The Alzheimer Page
www.biostat.wustl.edu/alzheimer
E-mail and archives

Caregiving/Support

American Self-Help Clearinghouse
Northwest Covenant Medical Center
25 Pocono Rd.
Denville, NJ 07834
(973) 625-7101
www.cmhc.com/selfhelp

Association of Jewish Family and
   Children's Agencies

3086 State Highway 27, Suite 11
P.O. Box 248
Kendall Park, NJ 08824-0248
(800) 634-7346
www.shamash.org/ajfca

The Carers Centre
The Vassall Centre
Gill Avenue, Fishponds
Bristol BS16 2QQ
England
CarersLine: 0117 965 2200

Catholic Charities USA
1731 King St., Suite 200
Alexandria, VA 22314
(703) 549-1390
www.catholiccharitiesusa.org

Children of Aging Parents
1609 Woodbourne Rd., Suite 302A
Levittown, PA 19057
(800) 227-7294
www.experts.com

CurryCARE
(800) 720-7440
Durable home care products

National Association of Area Agencies
  on Aging
Eldercare Locator
1112 16th St., NW, Suite 100
Washington, DC 20036-4823
(800) 677-1116
www.n4a.org
Information and referral to local
  services

Family Caregiver Alliance
425 Bush St., Suite 500
San Francisco, CA 94108
(415) 434-3388
(800) 445-8106
www.caregiver.org
Clearinghouse for memory loss and
  brain injury

National Association of Private
  Geriatric Care Managers
1604 N. Country Club Road

Tucson, AZ 85716
(520) 881-8008
www.caremanager.com

National Family Caregivers Association
10605 Concord St., Suite 501
Kensington, MD 20895-2504
(301) 949-3638
(800) 896-3650
www.nfcacares.org

Visiting Nurse Associations of
  America
11 Beacon St., Suite 910
Boston, MA 02108
1-888-866-8773
www.vnaa.org
Home health and hospice

Well Spouse Foundation
610 Lexington Ave., Suite 814
New York, NY 10022-6005
(212) 644-1241
(800) 838-0879
www.wellspouse.org

Further Reading

Dennis E. Kenny and Elizabeth N.
  Oettinger, *The Family Carebook: A
  Comprehensive Guide for Families of
  Older Adults*. Seattle: CAREsource
  Program Development Inc., 1991.
Wendy Lustbader and Nancy R.
  Hooyman, *Taking Care of Aging
  Family Members: A Practical Guide*.
  New York: Simon & Schuster,
  1994.
Virginia Morris, *How to Care for Aging
  Parents*. New York: Workman
  Publishing, 1996.
Virginia Schomp, *The Aging Parents
  Handbook: How to Take Care of Your
  Loved Ones*. New York:
  HarperPaperbacks, 1997.
Maggie Strong, *Mainstay: For the Well
  Spouse of the Chronically Ill*.
  Northampton, MA: Bradford
  Books, 1997.

Visiting Nurse Associations of America, *Caregiver's Handbook: A Complete Guide to Home Health Care*. New York: DK Publishing, 1998.

Web Sites

AARP Caregiver Resource Center
www.aarp.org/caregive

Caregiver Survival Resources
www.caregiver911.com

CareGuide Elder Care Locator
www.careguide.com

CareMedia
www.caregivers.net

Eldercare Web
www.elderweb.com

ElderConnect
www.elderconnect.com

San Francisco Examiner
"The Caregivers," by Beth Witrogen McLeod
www.sfgate.com/examiner/caregivers/index.html

ThirdAge Media/Caregivers
www.thirdage.com

End of Life/Grief

Canadian Palliative Care Association
(800) 668-2785
E-mail: llysne@scohs.on.ca

Choice in Dying
200 Varick St.
New York, NY 10014-4810
(212) 366-5540, ext. 242
(800) 989-9455
www.choices.org
Free state-specific living will, durable power of attorney forms

Hospice Education Institute
Five Essex Sq.
P.O. Box 713
Essex, CT 06426
(800) 331-1620, "Hospice Link"

Living/Dying Project
75 Digital Drive
Novato, CA 94949
(415) 884-2343

National Hospice Organization
1901 N. Moore St., Suite 901
Arlington, VA 22209
(703) 243-5900
(800) 658-8898
www.nho.org

National Institute for Jewish Hospice
8723 Alden Drive, Suite 652
Los Angeles, CA 90048
(213) 467-7423
(800) 446-4448

Further Reading

Larry Beresford, *The Hospice Handbook*. New York: Little, Brown and Co., 1993.

Ira Byock, *Dying Well: The Prospect for Growth at the End of Life*. New York: Riverhead Books, 1997.

Alexandra Kennedy, *Losing a Parent: Passage to a New Way of Living/A Guide to Facing Death and Dying*. New York: HarperCollins, 1991.

David Kessler, *The Rights of the Dying*. New York: HarperCollins, 1997.

Therese A. Rando, *How to Go on Living when Someone You Love Dies*. New York: Bantam, 1991.

Web Sites

American Academy of Hospice and Palliative Medicine
www.aahpm.org

Americans for Better Care of the Dying
www.abcd-caring.com

GriefNet Support Groups
www.rivendell.org/supportgroups.html

Hospice Foundation of America
www.hospicefoundation.org

Motherless Daughters
www.dfwnet.com/md

Palliative Care Council of South
Australia
www.pallcare.asn.au/

Practical Ethics Center
www.dyingwell.com

Financial

Council for Affordable Health
Insurance
112 S. West St., Suite 400
Alexandria, VA 22314
(703) 836-6200

Health Care Financing Administration
(800) 772-1213
Medicaid consumer information
www.hcfa.gov/medicaid/medicaid.htm
Medicare consumer information
www.medicare.gov

Institute of Certified Financial
Planners
3801 E. Florida Ave., Suite 708
Denver, CO 80210
(800) 322-4237
www.icfp.org

National Association of Insurance
Commissioners
120 W. 12th St., Suite 1100
Kansas City, MO 64105-1925
(816) 842-3600
www.naic.org
Free "A Shopper's Guide to Long-
term Care Insurance"

Social Security Administration
(800) 772-1213
www.ssa.gov/mediinfo.htm

Further Reading

Joseph L. Matthews, *Social Security,
Medicare and Pensions: The
Sourcebook for Older Americans.*
Berkeley, CA: Nolo Press, 1994.
Martin M. Shenkman, *The Complete*

*Book of Trusts: Everything You Need
to Know to Protect Yourself and Your
Estate.* New York: John Wiley &
Sons, 1993.

Web Sites

MediCARE Software
www.mindspring.com/tscotent

Housing/Home Care

American Association of Homes and
Services for the Aging
901 E St., NW, Suite 500
Washington, DC 20004-2011
(202) 783-2242
www.aahsa.org
Free brochures on housing, long-term
care

National Association for Home Care
228 Seventh St., NE
Washington, DC 20003
(202) 547-7424
www.nahc.org

Volunteers of America Inc.
110 S. Union St.
Alexandria, VA 22314
(703) 548-2288
(800) 899-0089
www.voa.org
Programs include affordable housing,
home repairs

Further Reading

D. Helen Susik, *Hiring Home
Caregivers: The Family Guide to In-
Home Eldercare.* San Luis Obispo,
CA: Impact Publishers/American
Source Books, 1995.

Web Sites

Ageless Design
www.agelessdesign.com
"Solutions to Living with Alzheimer's,
The Caregivers Guide to Home
Modification" (free download)

Continuing Care Accreditation
Commission
www.ccaconline.org
List of accredited retirement communities, consumer information

Homecare/Hospice in Cyberspace
www.ptct.com/html/industry.html

Legal

Legal Services for the Elderly
130 W. 42nd St., 17th Floor
New York, NY 10036-7803
(212) 391-0120

National Academy of Elder Law
Attorneys Inc.
1604 N. Country Club Rd.
Tucson, AZ 85716
(520) 881-4005
www.naela.com

Further Reading

Adriane G. Berg, *Warning: Dying May Be Hazardous to Your Wealth*. Hawthorne, NJ: Career Press, 1992.
Norman F. Dacey, *How to Avoid Probate*. New York: HarperPerennial, 1993.

Web Sites

Commission on Legal Problems of the Elderly
www.abanet.org/elderly

National Senior Citizens Law Center
www.nsclc.org

Nolo Press
www.nolo.com

SeniorLaw Home Page
www.seniorlaw.com

Long-Term Care/Facilities

American Health Care Association
1201 L St., NW
Washington, DC 20005

(202) 842-4444
(800) 321-0343
www.ahca.org

Assisted Living Federation of America
10300 Eaton Pl., Suite 400
Fairfax, VA 22030
(703) 691-8100
www.alfa.org

California Advocates for Nursing
Home Reform
1610 Bush St.
San Francisco, CA 94109
(415) 474-5171
(800) 474-1116
www.canhr.org

Further Reading

Sara Greene Burger and others,
Nursing Homes: Getting Good Care There. San Luis Obispo, CA: Impact Publishers, 1996.
Joseph Matthews, *Beat the Nursing Home Trap: A Consumer's Guide to Choosing & Financing Long-Term Care*. Berkeley, CA: Nolo Press Self-Help Law, 1993.

Web Sites

Horizons Group
home.algorithms.net/horizon/
Locates by ZIP code adult day
centers, nursing homes, home
health agencies

Senior Living Online
www.senioralternatives.com

Medical

American Cancer Society
1599 Clifton Rd., NE
Atlanta, GA 30329-4251
(404) 320-3333
(800) 227-2345
www.cancer.org

American Heart Association
7272 Greenville Ave.

Dallas, TX 75231-4596
(214) 373-6300
(800) 242-8721
Stroke Connection
(800) 553-6321
www.amhrt.org

Amyotrophic Lateral Sclerosis
    Association (Lou Gehrig's Disease)
27001 Agoura Rd., Suite 150
Calabasas Hills, CA 91301-5104
(800) 782-4747
www.alsa.org

National Association for Continence
P.O. Box 8310
Spartanburg, SC 29305
(864) 579-7900
(800) 252-3337(BLADDER)
www.nafc.org

National Foundation for Depressive
    Illness
(800) 248-4344
Referrals to local support groups and
    physicians

National Health Council
1730 M St., NW, Suite 500
Washington, DC 20036-4505
(202) 785-3910
www.healthanswers.com
"Putting Patients First," free guide to
    information resources for 170
    conditions and diseases

Parkinson's Disease Foundation
710 W. 168th St.
New York, NY 10032
(800) 457-6676

Pharmaceutical Manufacturers
    Association
1100 15th St., NW
Washington, DC 20005
www.phrma.org
Directory of prescription drug
    indigent programs

Further Reading

William H. Bergquist and others,
    Stroke Survivors. San Francisco:
    Jossey-Bass, 1994.
Rosalynn Carter, *Helping Someone with
    Mental Illness: A Compassionate
    Guide for Family, Friends, and
    Caregivers.* New York: Times
    Books, 1998.
Cheryle B. Gartley, ed., *Managing
    Incontinence: A Guide to Living with
    Loss of Bladder Control.* Ottawa, IL:
    Jameson Books, 1985.
Suzanne LeVert, *When Someone You
    Love Has Cancer: What You Must
    Know, What You Can Do, What You
    Should Expect.* New York: Dell/
    Lynn Sonberg, 1995.
*The Merck Manual of Geriatrics, Second
    Edition.* Whitehouse Station, NJ:
    Merck Research Laboratories,
    1995.

Web Sites

American Board of Medical Specialties
www.certifieddoctor.org
Locates specialists by geographic
    location and verifies certification

American Medical Association
www.ama-assn.org

Avicenna Information Supersite
www.avicenna.com
Free medical information databases
    search

Department of Health and Human
    Services
www.healthfinder.gov
Healthfinder searchable index

General Health Resource Index
www.achoo.com

National Institutes of Health
MEDLINE

www.nlm.nih.gov
National Cancer Institute
www.rex.nci.nih.gov
Neurological Disorders and Stroke
www.ninds.nih.gov

National Mental Health Association
www.nmha.org

Sapient Health Network
www.shn.net
Health news, bulletin boards about
chronic illnesses

Religion and Spirituality

Hanuman Foundation
524 San Anselmo Ave., Suite 203
San Anselmo, CA 94960
(800) 248-1008
Library of Ram Dass lectures and
workshops, books; catalog

National Federation of Interfaith
Volunteer Caregivers
368 Broadway, Suite 103
Kingston, NY 12401
(914) 331-1358
(800) 350-7438
www.nfivc.org

Shepherd's Centers of America
One West Armour Blvd., Suite 201

Kansas City, MO 64111
(816) 960-2022
www.qni.com/~shepherd

Spiritual Care for Living and Dying
P.O. Box 607
Santa Cruz, CA 95061-0607
(408) 454-9352

Union of American Hebrew Congregations
1511 Walnut St., Suite 401
Philadelphia, PA 19102
(215) 563-8183
(800) 368-1090

Further Reading

Zalman Schachter-Shalomi, *From Age-
ing to Sage-ing: A Profound New
Vision of Growing Older*. New York:
Warner Books, 1995.
Lama Surya Das, *Awakening the
Buddha Within: Eight Steps to
Enlightenment*. New York: Broad-
way Books, 1997.

Web Sites

National Council on the Aging
www.shs.net/ncoa/religion.htm

Spiritual Eldering Institute
www.SpiritualEldering.org

Reference Notes

Introduction

Often sandwiched between . . . *Fact sheet: selected caregiver statistics*, Family Caregiver Alliance. Further: *A National Report on the Status of Caregiving in America*, National Family Caregivers Association, November 1997: 71 percent work more than thirty-one hours a week, p. 5; 77.4 percent have children under 18 at home, p. 7.

Over age sixty-five . . . "Thirty-five percent of caregivers to the elderly are over 65. Ten percent are over 75." *Failing America's Caregivers: A Status Report on Women Who Care*, Mother's Day Report 1989, The Older Women's League, p. 3.

Three hundred percent . . . *Family Caregiving in the U.S.: Findings from a National Survey. Final Report.* Washington, D.C.: The National Alliance for Caregiving and American Association of Retired Persons, June 1997.

Chapter 1: What Family Caregiving Is

I saw grief . . . *Birdsong: 53 Short Poems*, by Rumi. Trans. by Coleman Barks, Maypop, 1993.

The typical informal . . . *Work and Elder Care*, U.S. Department of Labor, Women's Bureau, p. 2.

Similar dramas appear . . . Allan B. Chinen, *Once upon a Midlife: Classic Stories and Mythic Tales to Illuminate the Middle Years* (New York: Jeremy P. Tarcher/Perigee, 1993), p. 44.

If you think . . . Bernie Siegel, *How to Live between Office Visits : A Guide to Life, Love and Health* (New York: HarperPerennial, 1994), p. 5.

Access to care . . . "Growing APA elderly population adds urgency to improving health services," by Clayton Fong, *Asian Pacific Affairs*, National Asian Pacific Center on Aging, March 1998, p. 11.

Chapter 2: Women and Caregiving

Kore, the maiden, . . . Tanya Wilkinson, *Persephone Returns: Victims, Heroes and the Journey from the Underworld* (Berkeley, CA: Pagemill Press, 1996), p. 21.

To be strong . . . Clarissa Pinkola-Estés, *Women Who Run with the Wolves: Myths and Stories of the Wild Woman Archetype* (New York: Ballantine Books, 1992), p. 94.

Women are much . . . "Longer Lives: The Unique Role of Women in Long-Term

Care," prepared by the Task Force on Women's Issues of the American Health Care Association, 1993, p. 1. Further: "Exploding the Myth: Caregiving in America," by Robyn Stone, Agency for Health Care Policy and Research, 1987, document OM 92-00002: A third of informal caregivers report their health as fair or poor, with almost half of all spousal caregivers reporting fair to poor health, p. 20.

Women account for . . . Yvonne J. Gist and Victoria A. Velkoff, *Gender and Aging: Demographic Dimensions, International Brief*, U.S. Bureau of the Census, December 1997, IB/97-3, p. 3.

More than 50 percent . . . Kevin Kinsella and Cynthia M. Taeuber, *An Aging World II*, U.S. Bureau of the Census, International Population Reports P95/92-3, pp. 47, 48.

A quarter of all . . . *The Path to Poverty: An Analysis of Women's Retirement Income*, Mother's Day Report 1995, The Older Women's League, p. 1.

Older black and Hispanic . . . *Twelve Powerful Facts about Older Women*, AARP Women's Initiative fact sheet, 1994, p. 1.

A third of female . . . "The Income Status of Older Women," A Briefing Paper for the National Eldercare Institute on Older Women, 1992, p. 2.

Child care is expensive . . . *Failing America's Caregivers: A Status Report on Women Who Care*, Mother's Day Report 1989, The Older Woman's League, p. 1.

Although elder care . . . Ibid, p. 1. Further: *Work-Family Roundtable*, The Conference Board, Inc., N.Y., September 1998: In the next five to seven years, 37 percent of U.S. workers will be more concerned with caring for a parent than a child. From a fall 1997 survey.

Their health problems . . . "Caring for Our Aging Minority Women," by Jean Oxendine, *Closing the Gap*, Office of Minority Health, U.S. Department of Health and Human Services, June/July 1998, p. 1.

Fastest-growing segment . . . Minority populations are projected to represent 25 percent of the elderly population in 2030, compared to 13 percent in 1990. Between 1990 and 2030, the white non-Hispanic population will grow by 91 percent, compared with 159 percent for non-Hispanic blacks; 294 percent for American Indians, Eskimos, and Aleuts; 643 percent for Asian/Pacific Islanders; and 570 percent for Hispanics. *A Profile of Older Americans, 1996*, U.S. Bureau of the Census.

Although life is full . . . Jean Shinoda Bolen, *Goddesses in Everywoman: A New Psychology of Women* (New York: HarperPerennial, 1984), p. 278.

The old parents . . . Clarissa Pinkola-Estés, *Women Who Run with the Wolves: Myths and Stories of the Wild Woman Archetype* (New York: Ballantine Books, 1992), p. 453.

Letting live and . . . Ibid., p. 103

For most women . . . Ibid., p. 114.

Chapter 3: The Medical/Financial Maze

It is natural . . . Rachel Naomi Remen, *Kitchen Table Wisdom: Stories That Heal* (New York: Riverhead Books, 1996), p. 75.

I think modern . . . Elisabeth Kübler-Ross, *The Wheel of Life: A Memoir of Living and Dying* (New York: Scribner, 1997), p. 15.

The medical system . . . "Rachel Naomi Remen, Kitchen Table Wisdom: A Conversation That Heals," by Bonnie Horrigan, *Alternative Therapies* 3, no. 2, March 1997, p. 84.

Medicine has had . . . As quoted in "Looking to Illness for Enlightenment," by Georgia Rowe, *Contra Costa Times*, April 12, 1998, C9.

Long before there . . . Rachel Naomi Remen, *Kitchen Table Wisdom: Stories That Heal* (New York: Riverhead Books, 1996) p. 217.

To medicine's absorption . . . Sherwin B. Nuland, *How We Die: Reflections on Life's Final Chapter* (New York: Alfred A. Knopf, 1993), pp. 259–260.

The age-old covenant . . . "Physicians Asked to Renew Their Covenant with Patients and Society," Joseph Cardinal Bernardin Addresses AMA's House of Delegates, Washington, D.C., Catholic Health Association press release, December 5, 1995.

Healing is only one . . . David Simon, *The Wisdom of Healing: A Natural Mind Body Program for Optimal Wellness* (New York: Harmony Books, 1997), p. 5.

Chapter 4: Caring for Aging Parents

The ways of . . . Lynn V. Andrews, *The Woman of Wyrrd* (New York: HarperPerennial, 1991), p. 189.

We remain fixated . . . Joseph Campbell, *The Hero with a Thousand Faces* (Princeton, NJ: Princeton/Bollingen, 1973), p. 11.

Eighteen versus seventeen . . . *Ninety for the '90s: Painting the Future by the Numbers.* Illinois Department on Aging, June 1990, p. 6. Also *Failing America's Caregivers: A Status Report on Women Who Care*, Mother's Day Report 1989, The Older Women's League, p. 1.

More parents than children. . . ."Exploding the Myth: Caregiving in America" by Robyn Stone, Agency for Health Care Policy and Research, 1987, document OM 92-0002, p. 9, as cited in S. H. Preston (1984), "Children and the elderly in the U.S.," *Scientific American* 250, no. 6, 44–49.

Beneficial at moderate . . . University of Michigan School of Public Health survey, conducted by Louis Harris and Associates in 1992–1993. Study authored by Neal M. Krause. Report appeared in *Journal of Gerontology: Psychological Sciences*, November 1997.

Historically, in such crises . . . From "Caring for Our Elders" by Margaret Summers, *Essence*, December 1996, p. 22; quoted from her interview with Samuel J. Simmons, president and CEO of the National Caucus and Center on Black Aged in Washington, D.C.

The critical question . . . Naomi H. Rosenblatt, *Wrestling with Angels: What the First Family of Genesis Teaches Us about Our Spiritual Identity, Sexuality, and Personal Relationships* (New York: Delacorte Press, 1995), p. 351.

Chapter 5: Spousal Caregiving

Eighty-four thousand . . . Thich Nhat Hanh, from the Foreword to *The Fruitful Darkness: Reconnecting with the Body of the Earth*, by Joan Halifax (New York: HarperCollins, 1993), p. xiii.

We're the people . . . . "Spouses of the Chronically Ill Help Each Other Cope," *Journal of the American Medical Association* 269, no. 19, May 19, 1993, p. 2485.

The workload . . . Phone interview with Maggie Strong, April 2, 1998.

Usually our sense . . . "The Paradox of Finding One's Way by Losing It" by Michael Washburn. From *Sacred Sorrows: Embracing and Transforming Depression*, John E. Nelson and Andrea Nelson, eds. (New York: Jeremy P. Tarcher/Putnam, 1996), p. 195.

A patient heart . . . "A patient heart is the supreme means for transcending the suffering of the world. It is a shift from fear and grasping to letting go and forgiveness." Jack Kornfield, *The Roots of Buddhist Psychology*, Sounds True Audio, 1995, Side 5.

Chapter 6: The Nature of Loss

We must allow . . . Jack Kornfield, *A Path with Heart: A Guide through the Perils and Promises of Spiritual Life* (New York: Bantam Books, 1993), p. 180.

Known in Zen . . . "The Paradox of Finding One's Way by Losing It" by Michael Washburn. From *Sacred Sorrows: Embracing and Transforming Depression*, John E. Nelson and Andrea Nelson, eds. (New York: Jeremy P. Tarcher/Putnam, 1996), pp. 191-197.

Although this happy . . . St. John of the Cross, *Dark Night of the Soul.* Trans. by E. Allison Peers (New York: Image Books, 1959), p. 119.

The limits of self . . . Joan Halifax, *The Fruitful Darkness: Reconnecting with the Body of the Earth* (New York: HarperCollins, 1993), p. 16.

It is only . . . Sogyal Rinpoche, *The Tibetan Book of Living and Dying* (New York: HarperCollins, 1992), p. 33.

Grief goes in . . . Hope Edelman, *Motherless Daughters: The Legacy of Loss* (New York: Addison-Wesley, 1994), p. 5.

Adult life brings . . . Jack Kornfield, *A Path with Heart: A Guide through the Perils and Promises of Spiritual Life* (New York: Bantam Books, 1993), p. 174.

What used to feel . . . Sherry Ruth Anderson and Patricia Hopkins, *The Feminine Face of God* (New York: Bantam Books, 1991), p. 49.

Certainty of the View . . . Sogyal Rinpoche, *The Tibetan Book of Living and Dying* (New York: HarperCollins, 1992), p. 159.

The second journey . . . Interview with Sophy Burnham in *Sounds True Catalog, 1997 Holiday Supplement*, p. 3.

Dying is a mystery . . . Personal interview with Ram Dass, May 10, 1996; additional notes March 28, 1998.

Chapter 7: The Stresses of Caregiving

What is truly . . . Wendy Lustbader, *Counting on Kindness: The Dilemmas of Dependency* (New York: The Free Press, 1991), p. 17.

A study by . . . "Pessimism linked to more ill than optimism is to good" by Don Colburn, *Washington Post Health*, February 24, 1998, p. 5.

In a large survey . . . According to the *1991 National Health Interview Survey Report* by the National Family Caregivers Association.

Scientific studies show . . . "Why being happy keeps you healthy," by Dean Ornish, *Family Circle*, April 1, 1998, p. 26.

Caregivers don't live . . . Stanford University study results released March 27, 1998, United Press International.

Suggests Dr. Leonard Pearlin . . . From "Study Finds Elderly Care Stressful for Daughters" by Mark Evans, *Los Angeles Times* via Associated Press, April 12, 1998.

We must find . . . Jack Kornfield, *A Path with Heart: A Guide through the Perils and Promises of Spiritual Life* (New York: Bantam Books, 1993), p. 194.

Identify the emotion . . . Avrene L. Brandt, *Caregiver's Reprieve: A Guide to Emotional Survival When You're Caring for Someone You Love* (San Luis Obispo, CA: Impact Publishers, 1998), pp. 63–65.

Chapter 8: Caregivers and Depression

It seems that . . . Stephanie Ericsson, *Companion through the Darkness: Inner Dialogues on Grief* (New York: HarperPerennial, 1993), p. 69.

A headlong plunge . . . *Sacred Sorrows: Embracing and Transforming Depression*, John E. Nelson and Andrea Nelson, eds. (New York: Jeremy P. Tarcher/Putnam, 1996), p. 33.

More than 60 percent . . . *A National Report on the Status of Caregiving in America*, National Family Caregivers Association, November 1997, p. 8.

With a fifth . . . "Depression Alert," *Family Circle*, April 1, 1998, p. 56.

The dread and resistance . . . *Sacred Sorrows: Embracing and Transforming Depression*, John E. Nelson and Andrea Nelson, eds. (New York: Jeremy P. Tarcher/Putnam, 1996), p. 33. As cited in C. Jung, "Psychology and Alchemy," in H. Read, ed., *The Collected Works* (Vol. 12). Trans. by R. F. C. Hull (Princeton, NJ: Princeton University Press, 1994), p. 336.

The irony of . . . Ernest Becker, *The Denial of Death* (New York: Free Press Paperbacks, 1973), p. 66.

Average of sixty-nine hours . . . "An Exploration of the Plight of the Alzheimer's Caregiver," August 5, 1996, p. 3. Survey prepared for Porter/Novelli and Eisai/Pfizer, Inc., by Yankelovich Partners, Inc., New York, N.Y.

In a society . . . Thomas Moore, *Care of the Soul: A Guide for Cultivating Depth and Sacredness in Everyday Life* (New York: HarperCollins, 1992), p. 137.

The heartache and . . . Survey conducted by Consumer Health Sciences, Princeton, N.J., and the National Mental Health Association, August 11, 1998.

The best predictor . . . From E. J. Colerick and L. K. George, "Predictors of institutionalization among caregivers of patients with Alzheimer's disease," *Journal of the American Geriatrics Society 34*, 1986, p. 4938.

Beyond the physical . . . Ram Dass, "A New Vision of Healthcare," lecture at Disneyland, May 16, 1993, Hanuman Foundation audiocassette, Tape 2.

It's not always . . . Ram Dass and Paul Gorman, *How Can I Help?: Stories and Reflections on Service* (New York: Alfred A. Knopf, 1985), p. 195.

Eighth leading cause . . . *Fact Sheet: Suicide in the Elderly*, National Institute of Mental Health, 1991.

Rates increase with age . . . Centers for Disease Control and Prevention, "Increase in Suicide among Older Persons in U.S., 1908–1992," January 1996: People over sixty-five comprise less than 13 percent of the population, but almost a fifth of total suicides.

If the loss is . . . Connie Zweig and Steve Wolf, *Romancing the Shadow: Illuminating the Dark Side of the Soul* (New York: Ballantine Books, 1997), Chapter 9, "Midlife as Descent to the Underworld and Ascent of the Lost Gods."

A rite of passage . . . "Gifts of Depression: Healing the Wounded Soul," by Thomas Moore. From *Sacred Sorrows: Embracing and Transforming Depression*, John E. Nelson and Andrea Nelson, eds. (New York: Jeremy P. Tarcher/Putnam, 1996), pp. 214–222.

A life lived afraid . . . Naomi Ruth Lowinsky, *Stories from the Motherline: Reclaiming the Mother-Daughter Bond, Finding Our Feminine Souls* (Los Angeles: Jeremy P. Tarcher, 1992), pp. 57–58.

Despair is not . . . "The Paradox of Finding One's Way by Losing It" by Michael Washburn. From *Sacred Sorrows: Embracing and Transforming Depression*, John E. Nelson and Andrea Nelson, eds. (New York: Jeremy P. Tarcher/Putnam, 1996), p. 196.

Chapter 9: Hitting Bottom

Deep in the wintry . . . Clarissa Pinkola-Estés, *Women Who Run with the Wolves: Myths and Stories of the Wild Woman Archetype* (New York: Ballantine Books, 1992), p. 400.

The depths within . . . Jean Shinoda Bolen, *Close to the Bone: Life-Threatening Illness and the Search for Meaning* (New York: Scribner, 1996), pp. 29–32.

We cannot let go . . . Stephen Levine, *Healing into Life and Death* (New York: Anchor Books, 1987), p. 110.

Chapter 10: Support Strategies and Everyday Miracles

We have not even . . . Joseph Campbell, *The Hero with a Thousand Faces* (Princeton, NJ: Princeton/Bellingen, 1973), p. 25.

The fact that . . . Marilyn Webb, *The Good Death: The New American Search to Reshape the End of Life* (New York: Bantam Books, 1997), pp. 206–207.

Dr. Kenneth Pelletier . . . "Alternative Medicine for Seniors: Examining the Promise, A Conversation with Kenneth R. Pelletier," *Innovations in Aging*, The National Council on the Aging, Issue IV, 1997, pp. 15–19.

You are not helpless . . . Harold H. Benjamin, *The Wellness Community: Guide to Fighting for Recovery from Cancer* (New York: Jeremy P. Tarcher/Putnam, 1995), p. 12.

The role that . . . Michael Lerner, *Choices in Healing: Integrating the Best of Conventional and Complementary Approaches to Cancer* (Cambridge, MA: MIT Press, 1994), p. 16.

You are financing . . . Caroline Myss, *Anatomy of the Spirit*, PBS series. Also from "Anatomy of the Spirit: A medical intuitive looks at the emotional and spiritual causes of physical illness," by Caroline Myss, *Intuition*, September/October 1996, pp. 30–54; as excerpted from *Anatomy of the Spirit: The Seven Stages of Power and Healing* by Caroline Myss (New York: Harmony Books, 1996).

Mindfulness is vast . . . "Soul Work" by Jon Kabat-Zinn, from *Handbook for the Soul*, Richard Carlson and Benjamin Shield, eds. (New York: Little, Brown, 1995), p. 110.

Meditation is bringing . . . Christine Longaker, *Facing Death and Finding Hope: A*

Guide to the Emotional and Spiritual Care of the Dying (New York: Doubleday, 1997), p. 66.

Has the practice . . . As quoted in "Stephen Levine on Meditation" by Sean Meshorer, *East West Bookshop Catalog*, May–June 1998, p. 25.

Chapter 11: Caregivers, Religion, and Spirituality

The world was made . . . *Wrestling with the Angel: Jewish Insights on Death and Mourning*, Jack Riemer, ed. (New York: Schocken Books, 1995), p. 141.

When the dark grave . . . Joseph H. Herta, *The Authorized Daily Prayer Book* (New York: Bloch Publishing Company, 1961), p. 270.

While other things fade . . . "Why Stones Instead of Flowers?" by David J. Wolpe, *Wrestling with the Angel: Jewish Insights on Death and Mourning*, Jack Riemer, ed. (New York: Schocken Books, 1995), p. 130.

Go bury your . . . *The Aquarian Gospel of Jesus the Christ.* Trans. by Levi (Santa Monica, CA: DeVorss & Co., 1964), pp. 95–96.

If you would serve . . . Ibid., pp. 62, 63.

The highest seat . . . Ibid., p. 214.

No suffering, however dreadful . . . Sogyal Rinpoche, *The Tibetan Book of Living and Dying* (New York: HarperCollins, 1992), p. 221.

If we refuse . . . . Ibid., p. 14.

The path of life . . . Christine Longaker, *Facing Death and Finding Hope: A Guide to the Emotional and Spiritual Care of the Dying* (New York: Doubleday, 1997), p. 218.

Even as a . . . *Bhagavad Gita*, 2: 22–24.

Then I sought . . . The Eskimo shaman Aua, as quoted in Holger Kalweit, *Dreamtime & Inner Space: The World of the Shaman* (Boston: Shambhala, 1988), p. 145.

Did it make . . . Interview with Sophy Burnham in *Sounds True Catalog, 1997 Holiday Supplement*, p. 3.

The mystery of . . . Joan Halifax, *The Fruitful Darkness: Reconnecting with the Body of the Earth* (New York: HarperCollins, 1993), p. xxx.

Shamanism is a . . . Michael Harner, *The Way of the Shaman: A Guide to Power and Healing* (New York: Bantam Books, 1982), pp. xiii–xiv.

To the imagination . . . Alexandra Kennedy, *Your Loved One Lives on within You: A Beautiful and Inspiring Approach to Handling Unresolved Grief* (New York: Berkley Publishing Group, 1997), p. ix.

If we were able . . . Holger Kalweit, *Dreamtime & Inner Space: The World of the Shaman* (Boston: Shambhala, 1988), p. 75.

It is really difficult . . . "An Interview with Rabbi Zalman Schachter-Shalomi" by Michelle Bowman. Older Adult Education Network, the American Society on Aging, *The Older Learner* 6, no. 1, Winter 1997–1998, p. 1.

Chapter 12: End-of-Life Concerns

The spiritual labor . . . Marie de Hennezel, *Intimate Death: How the Dying Teach Us to Live.* Trans. by Carol Brown Janeway (New York: Alfred A. Knopf, 1997), p. 181.

The system makes . . . As quoted in "Last Passage: Can doctors learn to allow patients to choose death with dignity?" an interview in *People*, February 19, 1996, p. 87.

Stranger medicine . . . Christine Cassel, *All Things Considered*, "Roundtable Discussion on End-of-Life Issues," National Public Radio, November 3, 1997.

In a recent study . . . "The Quest to Die with Dignity: An Analysis of Americans' Values, Opinions, and Attitudes Concerning End-of-Life Care," a report by American Health Decisions, Appleton, WI, October 1997. Funded and prepared for the Robert Wood Johnson Foundation.

Several studies have . . . *Annals of Internal Medicine* 127, no. 1, July 1997. The Study to Understand Prognoses and Preferences for Outcomes and Risks of Treatment (SUPPORT) was first published in the November 22, 1995, issue of *Journal of the American Medical Association*. Further: More than half of seriously ill patients would rather die than live in a nursing home. *Journal of the American Geriatrics Society* 45, 1997, 818–824.

This study confirms . . . "Nature as Choreographer for Death and Dying" by Joanne Lynn. *Americans for Better Care of the Dying Exchange* 1, no. 2, December 1997, p. 2.

This whole notion . . . "A Conversation with Dr. Timothy Quill" by Sandra Beckwith, *Last Acts: Care and Caring at the End of Life* 3, Spring 1998, p. 1.

More than half . . . MetLife Solutions Forum on SeniorNet, August 1998. See www.seniornet.org/solutions.

A poll of doctors . . . N.Y. Mount Sinai School of Medicine study as reported in *New England Journal of Medicine*, April 23, 1998.

No matter how . . . M. Scott Peck, *Denial of the Soul: Spiritual and Medical Perspectives on Euthanasia and Mortality* (New York: Harmony Books, 1997), pp. 164, 165, 166.

The House of Lords . . . Ronald Dworkin, *Life's Dominion: An Argument about Abortion, Euthanasia, and Individual Freedom* (New York: Vintage Books, 1994), p. xiii.

Legal in the Netherlands . . . "Physician-Assisted Suicide and Euthanasia in the Netherlands: Lessons from the Dutch," *Journal of the American Medical Association* 227, no. 21, June 4, 1997, pp. 1720–1722.

In Australia . . . Helga Kuhse, "From Intention to Consent," in *Physician Assisted Suicide: Expanding the Debate*, Margaret P. Battin and others, eds. (New York: Routledge, 1998), p. 263.

Dying well is . . . Further reading: Ira R. Byock, *Dying Well: The Prospect for Growth at the End of Life* (New York: Riverhead Books, 1997).

To release our inner selves . . . Elisabeth Kübler-Ross, *Death: The Final Stage of Growth* (New York: Touchstone, 1975), p. 164.

One of the remarkable . . . Stephen Levine, *Who Dies: An Investigation of Conscious Living and Conscious Dying* (Garden City, NY: Anchor Books, 1982), pp. 249, 250.

When we're confronted . . . Phone interview with Dale Borglum, March 20, 1998.

Letting go of suffering . . . Phone interview with Stephen Levine, June 6, 1997.

There are no big . . . Carlos Castaneda, *Journey to Ixtlan: The Lessons of Don Juan* (New York: Pocket Books, 1972), p. 43.

The dying seize . . . Marie De Hennezel, *Intimate Death: How the Dying Teach Us to Live.* Trans. by Carol Brown Janeway (New York: Alfred A. Knopf, 1997), p. ix.

Chapter 13: Caregiving as a Rite of Passage

In the middle . . . Dante Alighieri, *Divine Comedy*, "Inferno, Canto 1." Trans. by Lawrence Grant White (New York: Pantheon, 1948), p. 1.

The dragon whose . . . Joseph Campbell, *The Power of Myth* (New York: Doubleday, 1988), p. 154.

Terror turn'd to comfort . . . Dante Alighieri, *The Divine Comedy.* Trans. by The Rev. H. F. Cary (London: J. M. Dent & Sons Ltd., 1937), p. 184.

The lord created . . . As quoted in "Sophia: Companion on the Quest" by Caitlín Matthews. In *At the Table of the Grail: Magic and the Use of the Imagination*, John Matthews, ed. (New York: Penguin, 1991), p. 119.

The soul world . . . Clarissa Pinkola-Estés, *Women Who Run with the Wolves: Myths and Stories of the Wild Woman Archetype* (New York: Ballantine Books, 1992), p. 421.

They appear when . . . Michael Meade, *Men and the Water of Life: Initiation and the Tempering of Men* (New York: HarperCollins, 1993), p. 377.

The deep well . . . Lorna Catford and Michael Ray, *The Path of the Everyday Hero: Drawing on the Power of Myth to Meet Life's Most Important Challenges* (Los Angeles: Jeremy P. Tarcher, 1991), p. 40.

A turning point . . . Dawna Markova, *No Enemies Within: A Creative Process for Discovering What's Right about What's Wrong* (Berkeley, CA: Conari Press, 1994), p. 52.

We are realizing . . . "Return of the Dark Goddess: A Conversation with Marion Woodman" by Penelope Kramer, *Intuition* 13, October 1996, pp. 49, 53.

There is a land . . . Thornton Wilder, *The Bridge of San Luis Rey* (New York: Grosset & Dunlap, 1927), p. 235.

So often we . . . "Begin the Adventure of a Lifetime: The Second Half of Life," an interview with Angeles Arrien, *Sounds True Catalog*, Summer 1998, p. 35.

In ancient times . . . Marc Ian Barasch, *The Healing Path: A Soul Approach to Illness* (New York: Jeremy P. Tarcher/Putnam, 1993), p. 75.

Those unfulfilled yet . . .. Gertrud Mueller Nelson, *Here All Dwell Free: Stories to Heal the Wounded Feminine* (New York: Doubleday, 1991), pp. 169, 172.

How can I . . . Trina Paulus, *Hope for the Flowers* (New York: Paulist Press, 1972), p. 75.

The toll for . . . Stephen Levine, *Healing into Life and Death* (New York: Anchor Books, 1989), pp. 70–71.

With no other light . . . *The Collected Works of St. John of the Cross.* Trans. by Kieran Kavanaugh and Otilio Rodriguez (Washington, DC: Institute of Carmelite Studies Publications, 1979), p. 295.

It is crucial . . . Michael Meade, *Men and the Water of Life: Initiation and the Tempering of Men* (New York: HarperCollins, 1993), p. 389.

The last deed . . . Joseph Campbell, *The Power of Myth* (New York: Doubleday, 1988), p. 149.

Chapter 14: Awakening the Heart

In daily life . . . "Your Grateful Heart: An Interview with Brother David Steindl-Rast," *Sounds True Catalog*, Winter 1993, p. 41.

Deborah Hoffmann . . . Phone interviews, November 29, 1994, and September 24, 1997. Excerpts: "For a long time" and "I'm very attached," *Complaints of a Dutiful Daughter*, Women Make Movies, © 1994, New York.

In undertaking a . . . Jack Kornfield, *A Path with Heart: A Guide through the Perils and Promises of Spiritual Life* (New York: Bantam Books, 1993), p. 11.

Chapter 15: The Urge to Serve

The characteristics of . . . Alice A. Bailey, *The Labours of Hercules* (New York: Lucis Publishing Co., 1977), p. 5.

There is hope . . . J. Krishnamurti, *The First and Last Freedom* (Wheaton, IL: The Theosophical Publishing House, 1954), p. 12.

Ultimately we shall be transformed . . . Ibid., pp. 286, 288.

Forms a life . . . James Hillman, *The Soul's Code: In Search of Character and Calling* (New York: Random House, 1996), p. 255.

We don't suggest . . . From "In Sickness and in Health" by Suzanne Mintz, *First*, November 22, 1993, p. 88.

This is not just . . . From "Yes, I Am a Caregiver" by Suzanne Mintz, *TAKE CARE!* 6, no. 3, Summer 1997, p. 10. Material also excerpted from phone interview with Suzanne Mintz, October 4, 1995.

Philip was my . . . Phone interviews with Elizabeth Sung, August 1996 and November 1997. Material also drawn from "The Restless Journey of Y&R's Elizabeth Sung (Luan)," *Soap Opera NOW!*, January 16, 1996, p. 5.

Anne Bashkiroff's mandate . . . Personal interview, October 1997, and phone conversations between November 1997 and May 1998.

I don't remember . . . From "The Hidden Problem" by Caroline Drewes, *San Francisco Examiner*, March 11, 1977.

When we came . . . From "Sharing a Private Tragedy" by Caroline Drewes, *San Francisco Examiner*, March 19, 1978.

If there is to be . . . Gail Bernice Holland, *For Sasha with Love: An Alzheimer's Crusade, The Anne Bashkiroff Story* (New York: Dembner Books, 1985), p. 176.

The highest service . . . David Spangler, *Revelation: The Birth of a New Age* (Elgin, IL: Lorian Press, 1976), pp. 199, 213.

Chapter 16: Caregiving and Community

We know that every . . . Elie Wiesel, winner of the 1986 Nobel Peace Prize, in his acceptance speech, as cited in Pesach Krauss, *Why Me?: Coping with Grief, Loss and Change* (New York: Bantam Books, 1990), p. 160.

The nature of aging . . . Ram Dass, recorded live at the Conscious Aging Conference, Omega Institute, New York City, 1992, from "Conscious Aging: On the Nature of Change and Facing Death," Sounds True Recordings, Tape A200.

Limitations and distortions . . . "Essay: Gerontology's Search for Understanding" by Robert Kastenbaum, *The Gerontologist* 18, no. 1, 1978, pp. 60, 61, 63.

Healer and sufferer . . . *Health Professions Education and Relationship-Centered Care*, Report of the Pew-Fetzer Task Force on Advancing Psychosocial Health Education, 1994, p. 22.

Love and compassion . . . Ram Dass and Mirabai Bush, *Compassion in Action: Setting Out on the Path of Service* (New York: Bell Tower, 1992), p. 4.

For it is not society . . . Joseph Campbell, *The Hero with a Thousand Faces* (Princeton, NJ: Princeton/Bollingen, 1973), p. 391.

Walk softly . . . Beth Witrogen McLeod, 1998.

Index